Feeling the strain

MANCHESTER
1824

Manchester University Press

SSHM

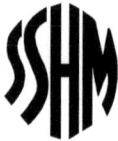

SOCIAL HISTORIES OF MEDICINE

Series editors: David Cantor and Keir Waddington

Social Histories of Medicine is concerned with all aspects of health, illness and medicine, from prehistory to the present, in every part of the world. The series covers the circumstances that promote health or illness, the ways in which people experience and explain such conditions, and what, practically, they do about them. Practitioners of all approaches to health and healing come within its scope, as do their ideas, beliefs, and practices, and the social, economic and cultural contexts in which they operate. Methodologically, the series welcomes relevant studies in social, economic, cultural, and intellectual history, as well as approaches derived from other disciplines in the arts, sciences, social sciences, and humanities. The series is a collaboration between Manchester University Press and the Society for the Social History of Medicine.

Previously published

The metamorphosis of autism: A history of child development in Britain *Bonnie Evans*

Payment and philanthropy in British healthcare, 1918–48 *George Campbell Gosling*

The politics of vaccination: A global history *Edited by Christine Holmberg, Stuart Blume and Paul Greenough*

Leprosy and colonialism: Suriname under Dutch rule, 1750–1950 *Stephen Snelders*

Medical misadventure in an age of professionalization, 1780–1890 *Alannah Tomkins*

Conserving health in early modern culture: Bodies and environments in Italy and England *Edited by Sandra Cavallo and Tessa Storey*

Migrant architects of the NHS: South Asian doctors and the reinvention of British general practice (1940s–1980s) *Julian M. Simpson*

Mediterranean quarantines, 1750–1914: Space, identity and power *Edited by John Chircop and Francisco Javier Martínez*

Sickness, medical welfare and the English poor, 1750–1834 *Steven King*

Medical societies and scientific culture in nineteenth-century Belgium *Joris Vandendriessche*

Managing diabetes, managing medicine: Chronic disease and clinical bureaucracy in post-war Britain *Martin D. Moore*

Vaccinating Britain: Mass vaccination and the public since the Second World War *Gareth Millward*

Madness on trial: A transatlantic history of English civil law and lunacy *James E. Moran*

Feeling the strain

A cultural history of stress in twentieth-century Britain

Jill Kirby

Manchester University Press

Published by Manchester University Press
Altrincham Street, Manchester M1 7JA, UK
www.manchesteruniversitypress.co.uk

British Library Cataloguing-in-Publication Data is available

ISBN 978 1 5261 2329 9 hardback
ISBN 978 1 5261 5609 9 paperback

First published by Manchester University Press in hardback 2019

This edition published 2021

Typeset by Toppan Best-set Premedia Limited

For Roy and Clare Kirby

Contents

Acknowledgements

Researching the cultural history of stress over the past few years, I have lost count of how many people have jokingly asked me whether doing so is stressful. While some elements most certainly have been, the whole experience would have been so much more difficult without the support, encouragement and freely given labour of many people.

At the University of Sussex, I would particularly like to thank Claire Langhamer and Lucy Robinson whose work and practice have been inspirational and their support unwavering. Sian Edwards has read and commented on various permutations of this research, providing insightful observations, good humour, friendship, encouragement and the occasional drama along the way. I would also like to acknowledge the many helpful conversations with colleagues, some of whom have shared offices, conference panels or worked on projects with me, and who have therefore also contributed to the development of this book. They include Rose Holmes, Natalie Thomlinson, Jessica Hammett and Laura Cofield. Special thanks go to Mark Jackson at Exeter University who generously gave me access to pre-publication sections of his own book *The Age of Stress: Science and the Search for Stability* and who has been supportive and encouraging of my work since we first met at the Stress of Life conference at Exeter in 2012.

Particular thanks go to Shannon Smith who has read and critiqued several chapters and whose clear, critical eye and scholarly but compassionate challenges have made this a better volume. She has also provided reassurance, support and cheer and, with Ann Hale, has organised and participated in several writing retreats whose atmosphere of sisterhood and collegial endeavour have greatly contributed to the book's completion. I am indebted to her scholarship and friendship.

I am extremely grateful to everyone connected with the Mass Observation Archive (MOA) and Sussex Special Collections, particularly to Fiona Courage and Jessica Scantlebury for their help, suggestions and generosity in sharing their knowledge of the collections, and to the board of trustees who appointed me Research Fellow for 2014/15, enabling me to finish my research for this book. I would also like to acknowledge the generous contribution of the many anonymous Mass Observers whose writings add so much to my work and whose insights and observations about life in Britain in the twentieth and twenty-first centuries continue to fascinate me and fill me with admiration. Material from the MOA is reproduced here with the permission of Curtis Brown Group Ltd, London on behalf of the Trustees of the Mass Observation Archive (© Trustees of the Mass Observation Archive).

Similarly, I would like to acknowledge my debt to the British Library and especially to the oral history curators Rob Perks and Mary Stewart in the Sound Archive, who have always been extremely helpful and informative in our interactions. I also want to acknowledge the generosity of the many people who have worked on the oral history collections and especially those who have given their time and their life stories in interviews, which makes this such an extraordinarily rich and valuable resource for the historian. I would also like to thank staff and archivists at the Learning Resource Centre at Roffey Park, the Wellcome Collection and The National Archives, all of whom were generous with their time and expertise.

Finally, as the research and writing of this book have been the focus of my efforts for some time, I must acknowledge the significant emotional labour performed by my family and partner during its production. Julian Ravilious has provided much needed perspective and, on several occasions, when I have bemoaned some tricky problem, cheerily suggested I give up the project, knowing this would jolt me back into sorting it out. He has also quietly and patiently always been there supporting me during the stressful times. My parents, Roy and Clare Kirby, have always championed, supported and encouraged their bookish daughter. I inherited my love of history from my Dad (though sadly not his encyclopaedic memory) and my desire to

communicate it to others from my Mum, and so this book is dedicated
to them.

Earlier versions of some of the ideas presented here have been
published as 'Working Too Hard: Experiences of Worry and Stress in
Post-War Britain', in Mark Jackson (ed.) *Stress in Post-War Britain,
1945–85*, Studies for the Society for the Social History of Medicine
(London: Pickering & Chatto, 2015).

Abbreviations

BBC	British Broadcasting Corporation
BMA	British Medical Association
BMJ	*British Medical Journal*
DSM	Diagnostic and Statistical Manual of Mental Disorders
GP	General Practitioner
IHRB	Industrial Health Research Board
IoD	Institute of Directors
MO	Mass Observation
MOA	Mass Observation Archive
MOP	Mass Observation Project
MRC	Medical Research Council
NCRIW	National Council for the Rehabilitation of Industrial Workers
NHS	National Health Service
PHC	Pioneer Health Centre
RGM	Regional General Manager
UMIST	University of Manchester Institute of Science and Technology

Introduction

In Britain stress is a dirty word. It's for wimps; a sign of weakness which should be not pitied but despised.[1]

In 1998, *The Observer* newspaper ran an article about Norwegian Prime Minister Kjell Magne Bondevik's decision to take a week off work due to stress. Under the heading, 'Stress just isn't British', it contrasted the sympathetic response to Bondevik's plight in Norway against the sceptical disparagement of British attitudes, dismissing his experience of taking time out for stress as 'not quite the done thing'. The newspaper claimed that in Britain, 'people who can't cope with the demands of work are perceived as weak. There aren't enough secure jobs to go round and anyone who admits to feeling the pressures and strains are scared they will be the next one to be made redundant.' Stress was therefore doubly difficult for the individual as it represented a failure to cope that suggested an inherent flaw but was also dangerous to acknowledge in a world of precarious employment. As a 'dirty word' it was best left unspoken or perhaps hidden behind the proxy of a physical ailment. As the language used in the quotation above implies, it was also closely related to understandings of gender. According to Cary Cooper, Professor of Organisational Psychology at the University of Manchester Institute of Science and Technology (UMIST), quoted widely in the article, 'Work in Britain is about being macho.'[2] This connection between work and gender identity made the experience of stress a threat to masculinity. It also ran counter to conceptions of work for both men and women in paid employment in the late twentieth century, which privileged endurance, competition and toughness. To find work distressing or difficult to cope with was therefore existentially problematic and for some simply too damaging an admission to make.

The idea that stress was something to be 'despised' also tied it to notions of shame and a sense that the individual was not demonstrating the stoicism that had been so closely related to notions of Britishness in the past and which continued to be referenced in popular media usage of terms such as 'Blitz spirit'. According to Cooper, employer attitudes were also problematic: 'Employers know they have a legal duty of care towards their staff but that doesn't mean they are wholly sympathetic to someone with stress. They'll do what they can only when it is in their interests. But understanding and accepting stress is another matter.' While those interests might be served by offering certain employees stress-management courses, the employer focus was firmly on making the employee resilient to stress, not on addressing what might be causing the stress in the first place. Cooper speculated that it was the British rather than Scandinavian model of work that would remain dominant. The article concluded on a negative note, suggesting that 'We can't stand people who feel sorry for themselves. This means those who stand up and say they are stressed are never going to be given an easy time. The future for our silently stressed workforce looks bleak.'[3]

The article illustrates the contemporary popular understanding of stress in Britain at the end of the millennium, but also the continuity of older ideas about work and mental health and individual weakness that had characterised the understanding of mental distress across the twentieth century. Popular ideas about who suffered from such problems were, until the latter third of the century, often closely aligned with status. So-called 'nervous conditions' were understood to result from overtaxing the brain, making them a problem of the educated and sensitive, and thus of the middle and upper classes, rather than the working man or woman. They also reflected dominant conceptions of gender that framed the domestic as feminine and the public, external world as masculine and thus tied ideas of causation to these domains. For much of the period, prevalent understandings of mental health focused on fears of madness and the shame of mental weakness and led to a culture of silence, privacy and extreme discretion, to the point that very often psychological problems were simply not spoken of or were hidden behind physical complaints. This tied causation to the failings of the individual rather than their environment or circumstances, thus ignoring any underlying socio-economic or institutional issues.

It was only in the last decades of the century that mental health issues and stress, in particular, became much more openly discussed and widely understood as the appropriate label for certain experiences.

The Observer was able to publish an article about stress without providing a definition of the term or explaining it because in 1998 it rightly assumed that its readers all knew what stress was. They did so thanks to cultural and societal transformations, particularly in the second half of the century, that had changed the ways in which people perceived and understood everyday experiences and their responses to them. Such responses included the way people recognised and dealt with the pressures and strains of work, but also the frustrations and distress of domestic and interpersonal relationships. Whereas earlier in the twentieth century there was a norm of stoicism and discretion, the latter part of the century was no longer characterised by the kind of 'Britain can take it' attitude mythologised in the popular memory of wartime Britain. These changes resulted in part from the increasing tendency to question everyday occurrences and to privilege the role of experts, arising from the burgeoning medicalisation and psychologisation of life during the century.[4] Such processes saw previously 'normal' experiences reinterpreted as medical or psychological complaints or as something that required expert intervention. At the same time, wider socio-economic and cultural change, encompassing contexts such as housing and gender roles, also contributed to the transformation of attitudes that problematised and increasingly made public, previously private or hidden issues. The media in Britain played a key role in popularising and emphasising this process, as The Observer article illustrates, particularly in the deployment of ill-health scare stories and increasing intrusions into, and commentary on, what had previously been private in people's lives.[5] Although Cooper acknowledged in the article that stress was at least now being talked about, the tone of the entire feature strongly emphasised the continuity of long-held attitudes towards mental health issues in Britain.

The writer of The Observer article could also reasonably assume that readers would recognise work as a likely context for stress and would perhaps share the underlying belief that it was the inherent weakness of the sufferer, more than the circumstances of their work, that was the cause of their stress. Although by the end of the century, stress *was* being acknowledged and *was* something that could be talked about, ideas about causation and who might be susceptible to mental health problems were often still firmly grounded in the past. This enabled mental health problems like stress to be understood as the problem of the sufferer rather than a result of their circumstances or environment, allowing employers, doctors and institutions of state to focus on the individual rather than the wider social, economic or structural issues that might be at the heart of the problem. *The Observer*'s reporting of the reluctant and often unsympathetic attitude of employers would also have been familiar, as would the sense of fear and insecurity about what might happen if the reader were to admit to being stressed themselves. Popular understanding of stress, as seen in media reporting, was, therefore, both complex and often contradictory.

For much of the century, mental health problems had carried a stigma and were something to be ashamed of, to keep private and to deal with discreetly. However, by the end of the 1990s, the ubiquity of the stress discourse meant that there was widespread awareness of the problem of stress, if not an equal willingness to address it. People were generally more inclined to be open about what earlier in the century would have simply been unspoken, and often unacknowledged, despite fears about the precarity of their employment. The combination of greater openness and a thriving popular, medical and institutional discourse of stress created an acceptance that life in late twentieth-century Britain was more challenging and complex than ever before. The apparent epidemic of stress that accounted for over thirteen million lost work days per year, was, therefore, an unsurprising outcome; and one that positioned stress as a significant economic, as well as personal, problem.[6]

This book was born out of my curiosity about how and why stress became so ubiquitous and whose interests were served by the ways in which certain forms of mental distress were constructed and understood across the century. It was also provoked by my experience at Birkbeck College, where stress was the topic for a term's study on a social science Master's degree, yet in the first lecture was roundly discredited as a concept. How could a subject that some academics in social science apparently disputed, be so successful and widespread an idea in other academic disciplines as well as in popular culture? Personal experience also raised questions about how concepts like stress inform our understanding of the self and the roles that gender, class and race might have played in the development of the stress concept during

the last century. Not all of those questions find an answer in the following chapters. In particular, race remains unexamined, in part due
to its absence in much of the source material, but also due to an
awareness of the potential intersectional complexities of stress and
race, which require a more focused research project in their own right.
This book is also limited to the British experience. Although there are
similarities between Britain and the USA and other western countries
in terms of how popular understanding of stress developed, there are
also considerable cultural differences, as demonstrated in *The Observer*
article's focus on the Norwegian prime minister. A comparative study
of stress in different countries would require a separate book, and
while there is some work that brings together different national
approaches, my focus here, as a British historian, is just on Britain.[7]

Most of the existing historiography of stress approaches the subject
from a medical perspective: the focus in this book is on both the lived
experience and the popular construction of stress, although elements
of medical and scientific approaches inevitably appear. In taking a
social and cultural approach and examining the everyday stress commonly experienced by the wider population, in this book I develop
our understanding of the ways in which people conceptualised,
explained and managed day-to-day experiences of strain and pressure
that eventually came to be understood as stress. In many cases, those
experiences arose due to the huge social, economic and political changes
to day-to-day life that occurred in Britain during the twentieth century.
As such, this work, informed by Alf Ludtke's approach to the everyday,
responds to omissions in the existing historiography by providing a
historical account of ordinary people's perceptions of daily life and its
stresses and strains, and the personal experiences of coping with stress
across different times, occupations and demographic groups.[8] It identi-
fies everyday meanings and traces the popular and vernacular discourse
of stress. In doing so, it not only examines how stress was known but
the ways in which that knowledge was produced. Drawing on a range
of sources, including self-help books, diaries, oral history interviews
and popular culture, my analysis foregrounds continuities in the
approach to managing stress and changes in ideas about causation. It
reveals a vocabulary of 'nerves' and 'nervous disorders' as precursors
to stress but also illustrates the mutability of the stress concept and
how its very imprecision gave it utility.

One explanation for the absence of historical work on the lived experience of stress is the challenge posed in finding personal accounts of stress. Often self-diagnosed, and for much of the century subject to the broader stigma associated with mental ill-health, stress has often gone unrecorded, and even unspoken. Ironically, the changes by the end of the century that made stress ubiquitous have perhaps also rendered it practically invisible and unquestionable except in its extreme forms such as Post-Traumatic Stress Disorder (PTSD). It has become such an inherent part of everyday life that we accept it as a given, brought about by a multiplicity of causes, unlike the extraordinary, singular events that frame trauma. While PTSD and many of its fellow psychiatric diagnoses are contested and questioned, the quotidian nature of stress has allowed it to permeate our existence, relatively unchallenged. This raises a number of issues that inform the approach taken in this book, including: the relationship between the meaning and validity of stress and its usefulness; the role of medicalisation, professionalisation and psychologisation in the popular adoption of stress; and attempts to explain its widespread acceptance in Britain through concepts such as 'affluenza'.[9] In the rest of this chapter, I examine these issues to provide context for the lived experiences and popular constructions of stress that I go on to explore in the ensuing chapters. This is followed by an explanation of the methodology adopted in dealing with the challenge of finding experiential sources and clarification of my use of terminology as well as a brief overview of the structure of the book.

Studies of stress

Early historical research on stress focused largely on military psychiatry and it is only in recent years that scholars have widened the field of enquiry. Key to the military focus was the idea of 'trauma' and the significant psychiatric impact resulting from extraordinary experiences labelled variously as shell shock, combat stress and PTSD, and about which there is a long and distinguished body of work.[10] This book instead looks at the ordinary and everyday stress that was much less likely to arise from traumatic or extraordinary experiences. However, public awareness of the psychiatric problems arising from the First World War undoubtedly formed part of a broader context of psychologisation and medicalisation that affected popular understandings of mental health in the interwar period and after and contributed to the way people interpreted more mundane stressful experiences. Similarly, the considerable public discourse and widespread understanding of stress in the later century enabled people more easily to grasp medical diagnoses such as PTSD. In exploring everyday stress and the evolution of popular understanding, this book, therefore, also provides a greater insight into the contexts in which more extreme psychiatric conditions became recognised and accepted among the general populace.

Scholarly works of history that have looked at non-military stress have focused mostly on the medical and scientific development of stress or have incorporated stress within a broader categorisation such as psychological disorders or neuroses.[11] There are two broad ways in which the history of stress has tended to be recounted. The first positions it as something that can be initially traced back to the sixteenth century and accounts of hardship and distress that were then linked to ideas about mechanics and engineering in the seventeenth and eighteenth centuries. These were developed and amalgamated with concerns about pressure and the pace of modern life in the nineteenth century, a key focus of which was the issue of 'overpressure' in education, particularly following the introduction of compulsory school attendance in 1880.[12] Sally Shuttleworth has argued that these concerns were an analogue of emerging industrial practices, and certainly these became the focus of twentieth-century theories about the effects of modern work and warfare on the individual.[13]

The second approach locates its origins more recently in the post-Second World War period, tied to the collapse of the old social order and as a 'potent manifestation of an unsettled and fragmented postmodern world'.[14] As Mark Jackson has suggested, a case can be made for both approaches. His own work effectively incorporates these two positions, charting both the medical and scientific development of stress over the centuries, and making a case for the very particular way that scientific studies of stress in the twentieth century have been shaped sociopolitically and culturally as well as biologically. He argues that our 'obsessions with the relationship between stress and disease' are a product of broader issues relating to the preservation of stability not just in physiological terms, but also personally and politically.[15]

Similarly, from a sociological standpoint, Dana Becker has indicated that the 'abstract and diffuse' nature of stress has enabled it to perform ideological work by containing much of our discomfort with societal change in the late twentieth century.[16] In most cases, however, both the longer historical view and the post-war approach have offered little insight into the lived experience of stress and personal accounts of experiencing, understanding and managing stress, which have been key to the development of the popular concept, and indeed to the huge increase in stress diagnoses.[17] This book addresses that absence.

As well as specific histories of stress, scholars have addressed topics which are linked to stress, some of which are mentioned throughout this book. These include suburban neurosis and urban planning; neurasthenia; revisionist work on neuroses in post-Second World War housewives and research into psychological disorders among men in the same period; examinations of work and stress; and the family and stress.[18] Again, few of these focus specifically on the experience of stress as part of everyday existence in the twentieth century. This book will address this relatively uncharted territory.[19]

What is stress?

Responses to modernity and change, and the importance of status, have been key factors in popular perceptions of stress during the twentieth century and appear as leitmotifs throughout many chapters of this book. One reason for this is the conceptual vagueness of stress and its forerunners. Stress and nerves have been available as labels for a range of experiences, have been interpreted in multiple ways, and have enabled the privileging of certain groups at specific times. Indeed, no research on stress is complete without an acknowledgement of the problematic nature of the concept: one that is, according to scholars across disciplines, 'so confused, to be almost meaningless' and with 'no precise or consistent definition'.[20] The following section explores the ways in which the concept has been explained, adopted, challenged and deployed.

As already stated, there is broad concurrence that the idea of stress originates in early understanding of engineering along with strain and was co-opted into biology thanks to the nineteenth-century view of the body as a machine, although there is some evidence of earlier vernacular usage relating to hardship and adversity.[21] However, stress as a medical disease appeared only in the mid-twentieth century. Ideas about homeostasis (the need to maintain bodily equilibrium) and the external forces which might put strain on the body (e.g. cold or heat) emerged early in the century, while in 1915 Walter Cannon's (1871–1945) book introduced the idea of the 'flight or fight' response, now commonly associated with the aetiology of stress.[22] However, neither this work nor the earlier ideas about homeostasis were specifically part of a stress concept. It was largely due to Hans Selye's (1907–1982) work, and particularly his publications in the 1950s that the idea emerged which would encapsulate not only the external conditions which might act as 'stressors' on the body but the resulting condition of stress which was the body's response.[23]

Tom Lutz and Michael Neve have both highlighted the analogous nature of stress and neurasthenia, particularly in terms of the size and value of the business created by both diagnoses and the cultural function that each has performed.[24] While readers of popular magazines in the early twentieth century would have failed to find mention of stress, Laura Hirshbein has noted that they 'could not have turned many pages before encountering some kind of description of nervousness or neurasthenia'.[25] This suggests that although stress was largely unknown among the general British populace until the late twentieth century, the symptoms and experiences that are now understood to constitute stress were certainly familiar. This is not to say that nervousness, neurasthenia and stress are interchangeable conceptually, but they do share areas of overlap and the ways in which these ill-defined, hard-to-pin-down concepts have been understood, operationalised and experienced were similar. Neurasthenia was seen as a disease of civilisation and modernity and associated with successful businessmen overcome by the relentless pressure of modern civilisation, as well as with highly strung 'nervous' women. There was status to be gained from being a neurasthenic. Lutz has argued that the combination of such a wide range of symptoms with these notions of exceptional refinement and sensitivity meant that it appealed to the elites who felt threatened by change and to the upwardly mobile who believed it would enhance their status, and this created an epidemic.[26] He has claimed that neurasthenia provided a vocabulary and shared cultural meaning that enabled people to perceive and explain the rapid change occurring in the late nineteenth century, and has argued that stress, being similarly available for plural appropriations, may have functioned in a comparable way in the twentieth century.[27]

The title of Serge Doublet's book, *The Stress Myth*, clearly set out his approach. In his book, he refuted the very concept, arguing that stress is simply one more in a long line of now discarded concepts, such as the vapours, hysteria, hypochondria and psychasthenia, and that it too may eventually be replaced by 'some newer and more exciting' idea.[28] He proposed that in biology, easily defined physical stressors are usually the main interest, and stress as the resulting condition is rarely defined or only in a generic sense. Something may be deemed a stressor by the 'mere presence of higher levels of stress hormones, such as cortisol' but he has claimed that many biologists, immunologists and virologists agree that stress is probably more complex than they assume, but prefer to leave that complexity to psychologists and social scientists.[29] Similarly challenging is Angela Patmore's view that 'stress is a mythical malaise based on an intellectual construct', and our fear of it creates the very condition itself.[30] Those working on issues of gender and mental health have also been critical, arguing that stress is used as an 'all-encompassing notion' to synthesise diverse distressing experiences and their impact on psychological states.[31] However, while acknowledging the controversy and confusion around the concept, Cary Cooper and Philip Dewe have emphasised its importance in significantly contributing to how illness is understood. They argue that if the durability of the concept is seen as a measure of its 'validity or usefulness', then this suggests it is worthy of further attempts at clarification.[32] This argument has had considerable support. As Lawrence Hinkle explains, 'there is still today no generally agreed upon definition of "stress" ... Nevertheless, biological, social and behavioural scientists have continued to use the term.'[33] Similarly, many other researchers, practitioners and professionals have also made stress the focus of their work, suggesting that a lack of conceptual clarity has been no hindrance to the concept's usefulness.

The usefulness of stress

Against such a background of conceptual mutability, there is a range of arguments as to why stress emerged as such a successful and widespread idea. Both social scientists and historians have agreed that durability and popularity might be the result of its very lack of precision, allowing it to incorporate a wide range of experiences and serve many different purposes, as neurasthenia did in the late nineteenth century.[34] A more pragmatic notion suggests that because the stress concept transferred easily between disciplines (e.g. from engineering to medicine to psychology and so on) it is in some way self-perpetuating.[35] Russell Viner has argued that Selye's stress concept found favour in two very powerful post-war groups, the military and industry, specifically because it appeared to justify their pre-existing ideologies (about combat neurosis and work performance, respectively). As a result, by the mid-1970s over one-third of prominent researchers in stress were based in US military institutions.[36] He has also argued that Selye was particularly adept at enrolling interests outside the establishment, so that by the 1960s the stress concept was also broadly accepted by alternative medicine. Although Jackson disputes the emphasis on Selye's role arguing that others in the field, such as Harold G. Wolff (1898–1962), general media and public interest also played a part, such a combination of networks of interest helps to explain the widespread acceptance of the concept at an institutional level.[37] The very easy way in which a diversity of experiences (of concern to different disciplines and interest groups) could be brought under one heading has also been suggested to explain what makes stress such an attractive and popular concept.[38]

The very versatility of the concept of stress and its capacity to encompass a wide range of themes has underpinned its utility and thus its persistence. For David Wainwright and Michael Calnan, 'the very fact that the category has such a powerful and persistent hold on both the public and scientific imagination suggests that it must at least partially grasp the reality of lived experience'.[39] Indeed Becker has claimed, in discussing how the discourse of stress has been used to locate women's problems within a medical rather than sociopolitical domain, that 'the more insecure a domain of scientific understanding, the more readily it lends itself to social uses'.[40] This malleability has enabled stress to be used selectively and contextually at both the theoretical and popular levels to support a wide range of ideologies, ranging from the nature of the social order and people's place in it to issues of autonomy and self-reliance and the reciprocal responsibilities of the state and the individual in health care.[41]

According to Ethan Watters, there is a popular perception that we 'invariably rely on cultural beliefs and stories to understand what is happening' when we experience mental distress. In turn, those stories shape the experience of our illness and thus stress, with its imprecision, gives us space for a wide variety of stories.[42] However, as Doublet has argued, stress may also be seen as simply the story 'du jour': people simply accept whatever explanatory labels are provided for their symptoms, and when new medical phenomena are introduced it is common to see a rapid increase in the number of cases diagnosed.[43] Again, the fact that the stress label covers a multitude of possible conditions and experiences has given it greater utility. In a more sweeping argument, Hirshbein suggests that the success of the stress concept is due to its implications socially, professionally and economically.[44] After all, whole areas of academic research have been dedicated to it, while within medicine, management, training and numerous other professions, stress has given employment to large numbers of people.

Medicalisation, professionalisation and psychologisation

Throughout the twentieth century, several interrelated processes have permeated everyday life in a way that has facilitated the development and adoption of stress. Medicalisation, professionalisation and psychologisation made it perhaps inevitable that by the end of the millennium, people would find stress a useful catch-all label for their widely differing experiences. Offering a psychological explanation, bounded by expertise and pathologising a range of previously 'normal' responses to everyday occurrences, stress offered a useful way of explaining people's reactions to the apparent challenges of modern life. The growth of stress as an accepted diagnosis for people's responses to the 'troubles of life', as Viner has expressed it, might be attributed in part to the increase in the second half of the twentieth century in a belief that professional guidance was needed to manage many aspects of our lives.[45] The role stress performs in different professions and networks of interest invites exploration of these underlying processes. While their influence is undoubtedly relevant to a much wider range of subjects than just stress, exploring how they have functioned helps to identify how understanding of stress has evolved and why it has persisted despite the debates about its imprecision and lack of conceptual robustness.

The medicalisation argument has suggested that medicine expands and develops new categories of illness in order to extend and legitimise the profession and exercise power over particular groups. Robert Nye has argued for a more nuanced understanding of medicalisation, suggesting that medical knowledge 'usually served individual rather than state interest' and that such knowledge sometimes works against medical authority as a 'form of resistance and defense'.[46] However, feminist writing on medicine, and particularly on psychiatric medicine, has focused on an interpretation of medicalisation as a tool of power and control.[47] A central feature of psychiatry has always been the development of new categories of mental illness, as they help to legitimate the profession's claims to specialist knowledge and expertise in care and treatment, and hence provide a *raison d'être* for those practising within it.[48] Evidence that would seem to support this comes from the Diagnostic and Statistical Manual of Mental Disorders (DSM), which is published by the American Psychiatric Association and provides the standard criteria for classification of mental disorders in the USA and, to some extent, the rest of the world. The DSM II published in 1968 ran to 134 pages but had expanded to a huge 943 pages by the time DSM-IV-TR was published in 2000.[49] Karl Menninger's pronouncement in the mid-1950s that most people had some degree of mental illness at some time, and many of them most of the time, undoubtedly reflected the growth in a wide range of psychological and psychiatric professions, and gave critics reason to suppose that psychiatry was making a pitch for the entire population.[50]

At the same time, the expansion of the 'professionalisation of personal problems' accelerated, exposing previously private domains such as the family and home to increased scrutiny.[51] Nikolas Rose has argued that the 'apparently inexorable growth of welfare surveillance' of working-class families arose from a complex interplay of the aspirations of professionals, the social anxieties of those in power and the political concerns of various authorities.[52] He offers the example of the 'complex apparatus targeted upon the child' that includes the child welfare system, schools, the education and surveillance of parents and the juvenile justice system. He has argued that the evolution of new professional groups to administer, regulate and manage such areas of everyday life thus created and propagated new forms of expertise.[53] That people accepted such expert intervention resulted from a dynamic driven by both economic expedience and the functioning of the post-1945 welfare state.[54] However, one consequence of this expert focus was to problematise many everyday experiences, resulting in a significant erosion of privacy and agency.[55] Similarly, the 1950s and 1960s saw the development of humanistic psychology that, as a reaction to the depersonalising tendencies of existing psychology, focused on the individual's potential for self-transformation, growth and freedom.[56] However, while focusing on individual self-development and potential, it also implied an obligation to improve. Against the backdrop of a society that increasingly saw the family and social relations as potentially problematic, this encouraged any individual failure to be interpreted as cause for professional psychological help.[57]

In the late twentieth century, this movement led to a more pessimistic understanding of the self, where self-improving self-sufficiency ceased to be valued, and the emphasis changed to valuing those who recognised that they were unable to help themselves and must seek help from others, such as the 'brave' addict who admitted their problem.[58] Coupled with a decline in social solidarity and political engagement, this enabled a therapy culture to emerge in which experts discovered a huge range of non-physical diseases and pathologised much of our experience.[59] A welfare culture that offered solutions through expert intervention rather than the self-sufficiency of the first half of the century, informed the exponential growth of this therapy culture which Füredi and Rose have characterised as more problematic than beneficial.[60] At the same time, both the anti-psychiatry movement and feminism brought mental health issues into the open and, coupled with the incorporation into everyday language of Freudian terminology such as ego, defence mechanism, and sibling rivalry, enabled the emergence of what David Healy has called 'psychobabble' in the media.[61] Such language, he suggests, bears little relationship to its theoretical origins and has harmful consequences for the way we view ourselves.[62] One argument contends that at its extreme, it is the very functioning of power by the professions, with the effect this has on privacy and agency, that might actually cause the very distress that then leads people in a vicious circle to seek professional help.[63]

However, the unspoken assumption of individual powerlessness that underpins these arguments tends to ignore the fact that patients can be active participants in the process of medicalisation. Nancy

Theriot points out in her work on medical case histories that patient testimony, as retold by physicians, can be valuable in illustrating the patient's representation of illness. However, as it is the physician who chooses which parts of the testimony to include, the account that emerges is not equally co-constructed.[64] A common thread running through the history of psychiatry is that it is practitioners who are under pressure to tell patients what they want to hear.[65] Thus, the knowledge and expectations of the lay population also bring pressure to bear on the proliferation of psychiatry and psychological conditions. Roy Porter, amongst others, has pointed out that this can only be because there are benefits to them buying into psychiatric or psychological paradigms.[66] Arguably, one of the reasons for the popularity of stress lies in the fact that conceptually it suggests that the distress we feel in everyday life is largely a function of our response to events, a response that we have the agency to manage.[67] Medicine is also not a simple, single entity and clinical medicine has been only one element in problematising life from a health perspective.[68] Among those other ways might be counted journalistic reporting of 'health' stories (or perhaps 'risk of ill-health' stories), particularly in the latter decades of the twentieth century, and the so-called 'disease mongering' of pharmaceutical companies who market diseases as much as the drugs they offer to treat them.[69] Another explanation for apparently exponential increases in mental health problems by the end of the century was that such problems were often hidden in generic somatic diagnoses in earlier periods. In the case of depression, Christopher Callahan and German Berrios have claimed that the preponderance at the mid-century and at its end was largely the same, and that the perceived explosion in mental health problems was not necessarily the result of medicalisation, but simply a question of labelling.[70]

The fact that people might deliberately seek specific psychological or psychiatric diagnoses from their physicians reflects another key historical argument that contextualises the emergence of stress: psychologisation. H. G. Wells (1866–1946), writing in 1924, suggested that the next century would be 'a century of applied psychology' and that there would be 'an increasing tendency to psychologise legal, political, financial and economic conditions'.[71] Wells appears to have been using his fictional time machine in being so perceptive in seeing where the contemporary debates about the mental hygiene movement might lead. The popularisation of psychological ideas really took hold in the interwar period through the creation of a practical popular psychology that owed less to Freud and psychoanalysis and more to an eclectic British interpretation of such ideas.[72] Indeed, in this book psychoanalysis features very little, mainly because, except for one or two of the self-help books examined, it was largely absent from people's experiences and therefore their accounts of everyday stress. Certain terminology entered popular culture, but although there was a surge of interest in psychoanalysis prompted by the First World War, there was greater support for a psychology of self-improvement than a psychoanalytic one of breaking oneself down. Psychoanalysis it seems had much less of a role to play in everyday stress than psychology in general.[73]

Although there is considerable debate about the extent of its impact, there is little doubt that the shell shock of the First World War created a heightened awareness of psychological ideas among the lay population as well as the institutions of medicine and government.[74] Mathew Thomson has argued that coupled with the shifting social identities resulting from increased leisure and economic changes, this encouraged the idea of self-improvement and the growth of psychology clubs and psychology as a subject for Workers Education Association classes and Trade Union education, as well as increasing usage of psychological concepts in the press and literature.[75] He has cited the example of the increasing willingness of people to air their problems through the advice pages of popular publications, quoting an increase in such coverage on the women's pages of the *Daily Mirror* from an average of 3 per cent during the majority of the interwar period to 27 per cent by 1939.[76] Support for Wells's assertion about applied psychology comes from the explosion in the size of the psychology professions in the immediate post-Second World War period when membership of the British Psychological Society grew from 800 in 1941 to 2,000 in 1960.[77] Within the public sector, clinical psychologists began to be employed in the 1950s and psychiatric nurses and psychotherapists from the early 1960s, as well as psychiatric social workers, while in the private sector a wide range of counsellors and other therapeutic workers appeared in addition to the existing private-practice psychologists, psychiatrists and the dwindling number of psychoanalysts.[78] This might partly be attributed to the growing sense that mental illness and disorders were much more common than previously thought, but can also be seen within the context of the discussions above about medicalisation and professionalisation.

Social scientific research in the second half of the century was significant in developing psychological approaches to stress, among them ideas about how psychological appraisal might mediate stress responses, theories about coping and about reactions to certain common life events.[79] The development of psychological approaches to stress sits within a wider context of the growth of humanistic psychology, focused on the individual's potential for self-transformation and in part giving rise to a boom in popular self-help.[80] However, it also reflects increasing industrial and organisational concerns about productivity and absenteeism.[81] Certainly, occupational stress became a particular focus in the interwar period due to transformations in the global economy coupled with changing perceptions of mental health that legitimated discussion about the management of the self.[82] Certainly, from the 1960s onwards, the history of stress can be understood as a story of expanding academic interest, particularly within social science, increased popular awareness and somewhat reluctant organisational recognition, as well as a rapidly developing 'stress industry' aimed at helping individuals and organisations to manage stress.

While arguments about the psychologisation of society in Britain in the twentieth century have recognised the medicalisation argument, they fall short of the sort of critical view that Nikolas Rose has adopted. He has argued that the 1950s saw a coming together of sociological, psychoanalytic and therapeutic expertise to develop theories about the strains of personality and human relations in modern life, in particular in the family and marriage, which only the techniques of experts could address.[83] Rose's arguments are inherently Foucauldian. He focuses on power and how psychologisation made it possible to govern and regulate people in ways that appeared to result from our status as psychological beings, and his views have much in common with sociological viewpoints.[84] Our increased valuing and privileging of autonomy and free will, while we are actually being constrained and controlled by it, is also apparent in arguments about the pathologising of many of the symbols of free will in late capitalist society, such as 'shopaholism' and 'co-dependency' and in discussions of the problematisation of alcohol use.[85] Rose has suggested that the psychologisation of society has led us to understand what people say and do only in psychological terms, almost as involuntary disclosures of the real person, superimposing the private on the public. Thus, public life and public actions are only intelligible to the extent that we can interpret them and understand them in psychological terms as expressions of private personality.[86] This psychotherapeutic context leads to an obsession with personal identity such that the self is defined in terms of how it feels rather than what it does.[87] At the same time, the pop psychology emerging from the 1960s enabled the creation of a whole new range of 'experts' who did not even need to lay claim to scientific data or clinical experience to be considered experts. Arguably it was this change that enabled psychology to become the underpinning ideology of the consumer society, propagated by advertising and market research.[88]

In the post-war period, increased affluence underpinned the growth of a society of consumers for whom happiness was always tantalisingly out of reach, embodied in the advertising and marketing of products they had not yet purchased. An apparent paradox of life in Britain in this period was that increased affluence did not bring with it commensurate happiness or well-being. In fact, some have claimed that it did quite the opposite.[89] Of course, absence or limitation of happiness does not necessarily equate to stress; however, the debates about why happiness did not increase with affluence offer contributory factors in the growth of perceived tensions and frustrations that became recognised as stress. The failure of material improvements in everyday life to deliver anticipated concomitant increases in happiness in the second half of the twentieth century undoubtedly begged for some explanation. For many people, stress provided it.

From an economic perspective, while affluence has freed people from subsistence living, it has not produced greater happiness. Well-being comes about through status achieved by comparison with others so that income relative to others is more rewarding than absolute levels of income, as is rising social rank. Thus, people become trapped in 'keeping up with the Joneses' in order to feel good and, as Richard Layard has pointed out, television raises the standards of that comparison because the more television people watch the more they overestimate the affluence of other people. We might apply the same reasoning to the burgeoning use of the internet at the end of the century, and to social media subsequently.[90] Advertising and marketing in attempting to win trust through a simulation of intimacy, devalued truth and trust, creating stress and reducing capacity for commitment and cooperation which are also key to well-being. According to Avner Offer, the new opportunities and rewards of market liberalism in the late twentieth century were unsettling to the individual psyche and saw a move from being a society of social equality, security and inclusion to one that was socially harsher and more business-friendly.[91] Despite greatly improved material living standards for most in Britain by the end of the century, the nature of the neo-liberal consumerist economy and society led to widespread feelings of tension and frustration and a background attitude of doubt and mistrust. In this context, the 'troubles of life' that might in previous periods have been navigated within a framework of stoic, collective support, were perceived as more pernicious and problematic than ever before and stress the ubiquitous result.[92]

Approach

While the preceding paragraphs have explored some of the wider arguments that contextualise the approach to stress in this book, the following section narrows the focus and explains the methodology I have adopted in historicising the experience and popular understanding of stress.

In focusing on everyday stress and on the experiences of ordinary people, issues arise around what constitutes the 'everyday' and the 'ordinary'. Claire Langhamer has discussed the ways in which the meaning of 'ordinary' shifted in time and context during the second half of the twentieth century, giving the example of how its loose wartime usage enabled the inclusivity needed to maintain morale. 'Ordinary' has often been used implicitly or explicitly as the counter to expertise or celebrity and often described what something or someone was not rather than what they were. She argues that while it was 'malleable and messy', the category of ordinariness particularly in the post-war period was also often used as a critique of expertise.[93] Ben Highmore sees the ordinary as encompassing commonality without 'necessarily intoning the ideological set pieces of "the silent majority" or of universality'.[94] It is this sense of 'not expert' and 'common' that imbues the approach taken in this book. Here 'ordinary' does not necessarily indicate working-class, as suggested by Selina Todd, but represents the experience of people who were not experts and did not deem themselves to be unusual or in any way significant. As Dorothy Sheridan and David Bloome found in their study of writers for Mass Observation (MO), people labelled themselves as 'ordinary' in opposition to other categories such as 'the posh' or 'the media', and it is in this sense that ordinary is understood in the following chapters.[95]

Similarly, in their work on everyday life in twentieth-century Scotland, Lynn Abrams and Callum G. Brown present the everyday as giving significance to the 'smallest aspect of daily life' through which we can extract an understanding of societal structures and values as well as the responses of individual subjects.[96] Their position sees lives 'shaped in the main by everyday practices rather than exceptional events', even in the case of potentially life-changing occurrences such as wars, and they argue that the repeated actions and routines of daily life are the background against which we define our memories.[97] This is consistent with Ludtke's description of everyday history as foregrounding the worlds of work and non-work and detailing ordinary existence through subjects such as housing, clothes, eating habits and 'memories, anxieties, hopes for the future'.[98] It is indeed some of those anxieties that form the focus of this book, and this stance on the everyday that underpins my approach.

Broadly, I have also taken what Porter expressed as the 'patient's view': I have tried to access the perspective of the sufferer and the people who tried to support and assist him or her.[99] Such a view, as Flurin Condrau has noted, is 'enigmatic' in bringing to light the experience of patients while also still engaging with them as constructs of the medical gaze.[100] Nevertheless, I have chosen this approach in order to reveal continuity and change in testimonies of stress and to uncover how stress has become part of our culture. However, my aim is not just to make visible the experience of stress across the century, but to examine the ways in which it has been constituted, particularly its popular expression. My approach sees experience as incorporating both language and the practices of everyday life and aims to situate and contextualise the processes, procedures and technologies through which knowledge of stress was produced.[101] As Todd has highlighted, people who took part in many of the social surveys of the mid- to late century were persuaded of the importance of their views and understood experience 'to be an important dimension of their lives – probably a more important one than the interior self'.[102] Therefore, it is the discourse of stress that arose from that experience, from the interactions between individuals and researchers, family, work colleagues, friends and neighbours, and that helped people to make sense of their lives, that I am interested in.

The approach has also, of necessity, been guided by the complex issues arising from any attempt to understand what people were thinking or experiencing in relation to such a sensitive subject as mental health. During the twentieth century those suffering experiences in this category often did so in silence or where they did seek help, it was in the informal exchanges with family and friends that went unrecorded or eventually in the sometimes illegible and often inaccessible notes resulting from a visit to their General Practitioner (GP). As such, sources for the historian of stress as an experience and as popularly understood tend to be fragmented, dispersed and inferred. Therefore, this book draws on a wide range of different sources in its attempt to locate accounts of the experience of everyday stress and to identify how understanding of such experiences changed over the century. Among them are feature films, self-help books, newspaper articles and readers' letters, personal correspondence, and oral history interviews. There is also a substantial number of reports and surveys carried out by academics, government departments and other professional institutions. While I have drawn on their findings, such sources are also indicative themselves of the topics of importance to the various sponsoring bodies at the time, and particularly in the post-war period highlight the growing incursions into the private life of Britons. At the heart of my research and threaded through this book is material drawn from the Mass Observation Archive (MOA). These sources provide insight into the everyday experience of ordinary people, and because they permeate so much of this work, I would like to offer some contextual information about MO materials and particularly those that I have drawn on.

MO was formed in 1937 with the intention of creating an 'anthropology of ourselves'.[103] Voluntary 'observers' were recruited to write direct accounts of their observation of fellow men and women, to write and submit diaries, to respond to regular sets of questions, known as 'directives', on an eclectic range of topics and in some cases to carry out bespoke investigations using a combination of surveys, observation and interviews. The volunteer observers who made up the panel responding to directives and providing diaries were a self-selected group, mostly from the lower-middle and upper-working classes with a tendency to be left-leaning. As Langhamer has pointed out, although representative of 'ordinary' people, they were in many ways extraordinary for the very fact that they volunteered their views and experiences and believed them to be valuable.[104] They determined what they contributed, which directives to answer and at what length, and this contributes both to the richness of the material but also its complexity and frustrations.

Replies to MO directives were analysed and the results collated into file reports. Diaries enabled the observers to record the everyday minutiae of their lives as well as their views and reflections on events, again to a level of detail and length of their own choosing. In many cases, they were directly addressed to MO almost as if the organisation were a person, and this meant that some writers revealed intimate details of daily lives, very often writing about things that were otherwise kept private and even secret. Such writing also encouraged a level of reflexivity that is particularly relevant when trying to understand private and individually constructed experiences such as stress, as it offers accounts and reflections that might otherwise go unrecorded. As the original founders of MO themselves were aware in relation to gauging wartime morale, the correspondents' writings gave a far more insightful response to challenging issues of feelings and emotion than the kind of answer given to strangers carrying out polls or other statistical research.[105] While not providing a statistically representative sample, the Mass Observers may be considered at least indicatively representative of people in Britain in terms of what they said about their experiences of stress and the culture in which stress was understood.[106]

While the original MO organisation eventually evolved into a commercial market research company and effectively ceased to carry out the same sort of social research in the 1950s, a new Mass Observation Project (MOP) began at Sussex University in 1981 and continues to carry out research today as a charitable trust. Material from this second phase of MO is based on the writings of a panel of volunteer respondents who reply to an average of three directives each year spanning a vast range of topics eliciting both contemporary comment and retrospective accounts. These have been invaluable in providing retrospective accounts of experiences of stress earlier in the century and in revealing the ways in which stress as a concept became adopted into late twentieth-century understandings of health and ill-health. Similarly unrepresentative, from a statistical perspective, the writings of the new respondents may be seen rather as offering 'telling' case studies, as discussed in Annebella Pollen's comprehensive examination of the debate about MO and validity, and this is how I have used them.[107]

A few words about my reuse of existing oral history interviews also seems pertinent. Drawing on recordings in the British Library Sound Archive that were made in the late twentieth century enabled me to explore life stories with the potential to extend further back in the century than would have been possible with new interviews. Those that feature as case studies in this book were selected because they all related stories of stress as part of much longer life histories, suggesting that these incidents had been significant to their sense of personal narrative, even if they were hardly the main focus. Oral history interviews, like MO writing, provide the historian with rich detail and in the case of life histories, allow a longitudinal approach that enables changes and continuities in one individual's experience of stress to emerge, as I shall demonstrate in Chapter 5 where I examine the account of Jeff Mills.[108]

Inevitably both retrospective oral history interviews and responses to MO directives that ask for reflections on earlier life require an awareness of the reconstructed nature of recollection. It is partly for this reason that I have not relied on only an oral or life history approach, but have used other sources such as contemporary publications, popular media and cultural products to enable some triangulation of the evidence. Recent debates about the reuse of data and, particularly, oral history interviews, have raised ethical concerns about the nature of informed consent.[109] Certainly, some of the interviewees whose oral histories I have drawn on were talking about their lives within a specific research context, for example about life in the oil industry, and thus my focus on their accounts of stress and nervous breakdown are unlikely to tally with their original expectations about the use of their material. However, I think it is pertinent that each of the interviewees chose to talk about their experiences of stress, usually in the context of their working lives, signifying that it was intrinsic to their life experience, although clearly only one element of a longer narrative. Researchers such as Joanna Bornat have argued that it is such fresh 'readings' of existing data which help develop new connections and insights, giving perspective not only on the past but also current understandings.[110]

Oral history interviews from the British Library Millennium Memory Bank, which were recorded and archived in the late 1990s in partnership with British Broadcasting Corporation (BBC) local radio stations, certainly enabled new insights and connections, as little has been published using or about these resources.[111] The collection was intended to create a 'snapshot' of Britain at the turn of the century and was based around sixteen broad interview themes designed to 'de-emphasise well-trodden topics such as war and work' and highlight change within living memory.[112] The collection's absence from much academic research may be due to misconceptions about the influence of the BBC's broadcast agenda on their content. However, these interviews are 'rich in participant-led narrative and detail', a factor which has enabled me to find in them accounts of stress which were surely never envisaged as key content during the original interviewing and recording process.[113] Therefore, by drawing on existing data within the British Library Sound Archive, I am able to provide a fresh reading of these life histories and what they can tell us about stress and its precursors in twentieth-century Britain.

Lastly, a brief comment on my use of newspapers and films, particularly from the post-Second World War period. Between 1918 and 1978, newspapers were at the heart of British popular culture with most adults regularly reading at least one national paper. This gave newspapers a social and cultural authority that enabled them to reflect and shape attitudes to everyday issues such as work and private life, both of which were pertinent to the development of the stress discourse.[114] Newspapers and cinema-going were also cited in some of the self-help books about stress from the early part of the century, as either causes of, or potential treatments for, nervous conditions, thus highlighting the sometimes confused and contradictory role of popular culture in representations of stress. Exploring these sources alongside life history and archival materials has enabled me to reflect the complex interplay of factors that led to stress becoming such a popular concept in late twentieth-century Britain.

Terminology

As discussed earlier, definitions of stress are problematic. In searching for accounts of stress, I have interpreted these sources and personal descriptions with some flexibility, particularly around the labels that people have given various experiences. The whole field of mental health, particularly in relation to vernacular explanations, is one of generic vocabulary open to wildly subjective interpretation. One person's 'nervousness' or 'stress' is another's 'deep depression' or 'nervous breakdown'. As Elizabeth Watkins has explained, 'Stress could mean the physical, emotional or social challenge faced by an individual; the body's response to one or more of these stimuli; or the pathological result itself.'[115] Therefore, I have taken in a wide range of terms such as nerves, nervousness, nervous breakdown, strain and pressure, and included explanations of experiences, which can be considered to sit on the stress continuum. Other historians have taken a similar approach in researching other mental health subjects, such as depression, or have incorporated a variety of specific medical diagnoses into broader studies of mental health problems.[116] Taking this approach has allowed me to draw on a wider range of sources, which in turn enables a richer picture of the lived experiences of stress and nervous suffering to emerge. I align myself with Watkins, who has written about how, when and why stress entered the American vernacular. Like her, I do not attempt to offer a precise definition of stress but am more interested in how the very imprecision of concepts like stress and its predecessors allowed them to be deployed in a wide range of circumstances by different people.[117]

At its heart, this book tracks this popular usage and the changes and continuities of its deployment over the century. I do this by looking at people's attitudes and responses towards their experiences of the 'troubles of life', which were recorded under several different labels during the twentieth century, some of which fell within specific contemporary medical diagnostic categories and some of which might now be identified quite differently.[118] Diagnostic categories are historically specific and arise from particular medical, social, economic, institutional and cultural conditions. Indeed, the context for Selye's development of the stress concept is addressed in some detail in Jackson's book on stress, but my point is that such is the mutability of many mental health constructs that historians of conditions as varied as depression, nervous breakdown and stress might all plough the same research ground with equal justification.[119]

Similarly, it has not been my intention to retro-diagnose the individuals who emerge from my sources, so as much as possible I adopt their terminology, reserving 'stress' as the label for the generic, overarching concept or where it is the appropriate contemporary term in the later century. Therefore, for much of the book what is revealed in the newspapers, diaries, survey responses, self-help books, films and television programmes, which form its main sources, is a lexicon of nerves that includes 'nervous conditions', 'nervous breakdown', 'nervous exhaustion', 'neurasthenia' and various other expressions. That such terms were extremely flexible and understood to be so, was highlighted by Richard Asher, a physician at the Central Middlesex Hospital, in his 1957 self-help book *Nerves Explained*. He commented, 'if somebody says a relation has had a nervous breakdown it may mean they have been insane or it may only mean they have had a mild nervous upset'.[120] I have accepted the descriptions and labels provided in the sources I have studied, and effectively use the explanations of the experiences that they reveal to decide on whether they fit within the very broad and elastic popular conception of nerves and/or stress in any particular period.

Map of the book

The structure of the book is chronological and in the first chapter I examine self-help literature from the early twentieth century and establish some of the ways in which popular understanding of issues affecting mental well-being were explained, the terminology used and the treatments and remedies suggested. While self-help books do not access the experience of stress per se, they do provide a starting point for understanding what explanations were available at a popular level for those suffering various forms of nervous distress. These books offer insights into understandings of nerves, which is the term most frequently used in the texts, as they relied solely on the reader's self-diagnosis, and addressed issues that sufferers may have been reluctant or unable to deal with within the formal framework of institutional medicine. They represent the opening up of a discourse about the inner self and the sensitive area of mental health and illustrate the increasing reflexivity required to explain everyday life in the twentieth century. However, at the same time, they were a discreet remedy that enabled readers to avoid the reification of their concerns through formal medical diagnosis or the prognostications of experts. Self-help literature reflected and responded to contemporary social problems, highlighting enduring human concerns and changing social needs. It also contributed to that social change, as it not only reflected concerns but also offered explicit instructions on how to deal with them, revealing a construction of nervous illness influenced by both gender and class. Self-help books were also illustrative of popular notions of health and well-being, stoicism and personal responsibility. This chapter lays the groundwork for succeeding chapters in establishing popular understandings of causation and treatment and revealing the considerable flexibility inherent within the overall concept of nerves.

Chapter 2 explores how the experience of stress was interpreted within two very different contexts: the workplace and the home. First, by critically engaging with contemporary research into employee neurosis in the interwar period, I illustrate attitudes towards work, duty and responsibility. I argue that the role of work in the construction of personal identity, and social and economic life contributed to the difficulty of admitting to nervous problems and to a stoicism that meant people simply endured whatever mental suffering arose, whether at work or at home. Second, I argue that employer attitudes to stress revealed in this research, focusing on its impact on productivity and a desire to identify those who might be susceptible to it, established a pattern that underpinned organisational approaches to stress for most of the century. An examination of how similar concerns about neuroticism were applied within the domestic context through the development of Dr Stephen Taylor's (1910–1988) suburban neurosis diagnosis and work carried out by the Pioneer Health Centre in Peckham in the 1930s and 1940s, reveals how domestic stress was gendered but also how changing conceptions of the home and burgeoning social mobility fuelled understandings of stress.

In Chapter 3, which focuses on the Second World War, early unsubstantiated government concerns about the psychiatric impact of bombing on the population are contrasted with the experience of civilian stress that arose largely from the daily strain of wartime living and the specific demands made of workers in a wartime economy. In doing so, I draw attention to the gendered nature of stress, particularly how the conscripted female workforce responded to the challenges of disrupted and difficult domestic lives as well as the expectations of employers. I argue that one of the few ways women had of establishing agency was through the high levels of absenteeism that so worried employers and the wartime government. While projects such as Roffey Park Rehabilitation Centre and the work of organisational Welfare Officers reveal recognition of employee suffering and attempts to deal with it, they were also grounded in concerns about production and, against a backdrop of expected collective wartime stoicism, were based on assumptions about individual, inherent weakness as the cause of stress.

Chapter 4 charts the ways in which social change experienced through housing and gender roles enabled domestic stress to become more visible. Initially focused on the wartime case study of Mrs C and her troubled marriage, the chapter examines interpersonal relationships and sites of domestic contestation around control of time and resources. Changing conceptualisations of the home, and growing expectations of privacy and material comfort in the post-war period, led to increasing mental distress, particularly when material circumstances did not live up to those expectations. The chapter also highlights the tensions arising from the home being their workplace for most women. It offers evidence both to support and counter recent revisionist accounts of the role of domestic work in women's experiences of anxiety and depression.[121] In doing so, it reveals how the complexities and contradictions of such work gave the home more prominence as a potential location and cause of stress. The breakdown of tightly knit, stable communities in the second half of the century also provides the context for an increase in perceived stress. The way in which this was then portrayed in popular culture, such as the New Wave 'kitchen-sink' dramas of the late 1950s and early 1960s, both reflected and helped to construct people's experience of stress.

Chapter 5 focuses on change and continuity in popular conceptions of stress and status in the 1960s and 1970s, and how the public, popular discourse of stress increasingly revealed in newspaper reporting shifted from positioning stress as a workplace problem of the managerial class to a label that could be placed on almost anyone, in any circumstances at any stage in their life. As such I highlight the way in which the concept of stress was both gendered and class-specific and why this changed during this period. Placed in contrast to this increasing public discourse is the examination of three case studies of individual accounts of work stress in the early 1970s. These suggest the relatively limited impact of the public discourse on the way that individuals interpreted their own experiences and the responses to their suffering from colleagues and the medical profession. They represent considerable continuity with earlier explanations which privileged physical symptoms, and which focused on the individual's weakness rather than the contribution of the environmental or social context of the workplace. This time lag between the popular discourse and personal interpretations of experience implies that the 1970s was effectively the transition decade before the culture of stress became truly normalised in British society.

Chapter 6 examines the effects of the increased public stress discourse, with particular reference to organisational responses. The way that employers responded to the growing problem of stress revealed continuity in terms of the contingent approach to, and explanation of, employee stress as a problem of the individual, rather than an environmental or organisational one. Popular representations of the stressed and the development of ideas about 'burn-out' also highlighted continuities with previous attempts to categorise those most susceptible to stress and reveal links between status and people's attitudes not just to their work but to the changing economic and social context of Britain at the end of the twentieth century. This continued focus on the idea of stress and its institutionalisation within work and domestic life also played into an increasing conceptualisation of the individual as victim. While, on the one hand, this liberated the stress sufferer from being the cause of their own suffering, it also removed their agency to address the problem and still to some extent implied a level of personal weakness, consistent with the conceptualisation of stress throughout the century.

At the heart of this book is the argument that despite material improvements in both work and home life during the twentieth century, societal changes and a growing popular discourse of stress meant that by the end of the millennium, people regularly interpreted their everyday woes as stress. Alongside this, it shows how before stress emerged as a recognised medical diagnosis at the mid-century, many of the experiences that we might now understand as stress existed and were

articulated through the language of nerves and nervousness. That
language and the terminology that people employed to describe their
experiences were largely historicised according to cultural and social
acceptability. Thus, physical explanations and understandings were
privileged for much of the century, and both class and gender influenced
explanations of causation and proposed treatments. For much of the
early part of the century, material circumstances, economic necessity
and the agency of a survivalist approach ensured that any stressful
experiences were likely to go unacknowledged, as stoicism was popularly
understood as the appropriate response. It was changes in the ways
that people understood their everyday experiences of work and domestic
life and the strategies they used to manage them, particularly in the
post-Second World War period, thanks to increasing education, affluence
and consumerism, that led to such experiences being both problematised
and the concept of stress popularised. What *Feeling the strain* illustrates
is how a mutable concept like stress can be useful to a range of stakeholders, its multivalency ensuring both longevity and, by the end of the
twentieth century, the ubiquity of stress.

Notes

1 'Stress Just Isn't British', *Observer*, 6 September 1998, p. 12.
2 *Ibid.*
3 *Ibid.*
4 For an account of the process of psychologisation in Britain during the
  twentieth century, see Mathew Thomson, *Psychological Subjects: Identity,
  Culture, and Health in Twentieth-Century Britain* (Oxford: Oxford
  University Press, 2006).
5 For an examination of the evolution of sexual content and intrusion
  into private lives in the popular press, see Adrian Bingham, *Family
  Newspapers? Sex, Private Life and the British Popular Press 1918–1978*
  (Oxford: Oxford University Press, 2009).
6 National Statistics, 'Health and Safety Commission Highlights 2001/2'
  (Health and Safety Executive, 2002), p. 6, www.hse.gov.uk/statistics/
  overall/hssh0102.pdf?pdf=hssh0102. Accessed 12 November 2017.
7 David Cantor and Edmund Ramsden (eds), *Stress, Shock, and Adaptation
  in the Twentieth Century* (Rochester, NY: University of Rochester Press,
  2014). Includes chapters on stress in Britain, the USA and Japan.
8 Lynn Abrams and Callum G. Brown, *A History of Everyday Life in
  Twentieth-Century Scotland* (Edinburgh: Edinburgh University Press,

2010); Ben Highmore, *Everyday Life and Cultural Theory: An Introduction* (London: Routledge, 2002); Claire Langhamer, "'Who the Hell Are Ordinary People?" Ordinariness as a Category of Historical Analysis', *Transactions of the Royal Historical Society* 28 (2018).

9 Oliver James, *Affluenza* (London: Vermilion, 2007). James defines affluenza as a condition of the twenty-first-century obsessive, envious, competitive middle class which makes people prone to depression, anxiety and addictions.

10 See for example: Edgar Jones, *Shell Shock to PTSD: Military Psychiatry from 1900 to the Gulf War* (Hove; New York: Psychology Press, 2005); Ben Shephard, *A War of Nerves: Soldiers and Psychiatrists in the Twentieth Century* (Cambridge, MA: Harvard University Press, 2001); Allan Young, *The Harmony of Illusions: Inventing Post-Traumatic Stress Disorder* (Princeton; Chichester: Princeton University Press, 1995); Harold Merskey, 'Post-Traumatic Stress Disorder and Shell Shock: Clinical Section', in German Elias Berrios and Roy Porter (eds) *A History of Clinical Psychiatry: The Origin and History of Psychiatric Disorders* (London: The Athlone Press, 1995); Jo Stanley, 'Involuntary Commemorations', in T. G. Ashplant, Graham Dawson and Michael Roper (eds) *The Politics of War Memory and Commemoration* (London: Routledge, 2000); Derek Summerfield, 'The Invention of Post-Traumatic Stress Disorder and the Social Usefulness of a Psychiatric Category', *BMJ* 322 (2001); Peter Barham, *Forgotten Lunatics of the Great War* (New Haven; London: Yale University Press, 2004).

11 Mark Jackson, *The Age of Stress: Science and the Search for Stability* (Oxford: Oxford University Press, 2013); Ali Haggett, *Desperate Housewives, Neuroses and the Domestic Environment, 1945–1970* (London: Pickering & Chatto, 2012); Ali Haggett, *A History of Male Psychological Disorders in Britain, 1945–1970* (Basingstoke: Palgrave Macmillan, 2015).

12 J. Middleton, 'The Overpressure Epidemic of 1884 and the Culture of Nineteenth-Century Schooling', *History of Education* 33, 4 (July 2004): p. 420, https://doi.org/10.1080/0046760042000221808.

13 Sally Shuttleworth, *The Mind of the Child: Child Development in Literature, Science, and Medicine, 1840–1900* (Oxford: Oxford University Press, 2010), p. 140; Cary L. Cooper and Philip Dewe, *Stress: A Brief History* (Oxford: Blackwell, 2004), pp. 1–7.

14 Mark Jackson, 'Stress in Post-War Britain: An Introduction', in Mark Jackson (ed.) *Stress in Post-War Britain, 1945–85*, Studies for the Society for the Social History of Medicine 23 (London: Pickering & Chatto, 2015), pp. 5–6.

15 *Ibid.*, p. 7.
16 Dana Becker, *One Nation Under Stress: The Trouble with Stress as an Idea* (Oxford: Oxford University Press, 2013), p. 17.
17 Jackson, *Age of Stress*; Mark Jackson, 'Am I Ill?' (Illness Histories and Approaches Workshop, History Department, King's College London, 2012).
18 Rhodri Hayward, 'Desperate Housewives and Model Amoebae: The Invention of Suburban Neurosis in Inter-War Britain', in Mark Jackson (ed.) *Health and the Modern Home* (New York: Routledge, 2007); Edmund Ramsden, 'Stress in the City: Mental Health, Urban Planning, and the Social Sciences in the Postwar United States', in Cantor and Ramsden (eds) *Stress, Shock, and Adaptation*; Mathew Thomson, 'Neurasthenia in Britain: An Overview', in Marijke Gijswijt-Hofstra and Roy Porter (eds) *Cultures of Psychiatry and Mental Health Care in Postwar Britain and the Netherlands*, Clio Medica / The Wellcome Series in the History of Medicine (Amsterdam: Rodopi, 2001); Haggett, *Desperate Housewives*; Haggett, *Male Psychological Disorders*; Sarah Hayes, 'Industrial Automation and Stress, c. 1945–79', in Jackson (ed.) *Stress in Post-War Britain*; Joseph Melling, 'Labouring Stress: Scientific Research, Trade Unions and Perceptions of Workplace Stress in Mid-Twentieth Century Britain', in Jackson (ed.) *Stress in Post-War Britain*; Joseph Melling, 'Making Sense of Workplace Fear: The Role of Physicians, Psychiatrists, and Labor in Reforming Occupational Strain in Industrial Britain, ca. 1850–1970', in Cantor and Ramsden (eds) *Stress, Shock, and Adaptation*; Debbie Palmer, 'Cultural Change, Stress and Civil Servants' Occupational Health, c. 1967–85', in Jackson (ed.) *Stress in Post-War Britain*; Pamela Richardson, 'From War to Peace: Families Adapting to Change', in Mark Jackson (ed.) *Stress in Post-War Britain*; Nicole Baur, 'Families, Stress and Mental Illness in Devon, 1940s to 1970s', in Jackson (ed.) *Stress in Post-War Britain*.
19 Works which do engage with personal experience include: Richardson, 'From War to Peace'; Baur, 'Families'; Haggett, *Desperate Housewives*.
20 Cooper and Dewe, *Stress*, pp. 110–11. Jackson, *Age of Stress*, p. 1. Indeed Patmore includes a whole chapter about the problematic nature of its definition in Angela Patmore, *The Truth about Stress* (London: Atlantic, 2006).
21 Jackson, *Age of Stress*, p. 37; Cooper and Dewe, *Stress*, pp. 3–5.
22 Jackson, *Age of Stress*, p. 11. Walter Bradford Cannon, *Bodily Changes in Pain, Hunger, Fear and Rage: An Account of Recent Researches into the Function of Emotional Excitement* (New York; London: D. Appleton and Co., 1915), p. 187.

23 Hans Selye, *The Stress of Life* (New York: McGraw-Hill, 1956).

24 Tom Lutz, 'Neurasthenia and Fatigue Syndromes: Social Section', in German Elias Berrios and Roy Porter (eds) *A History of Clinical Psychiatry*, p. 542; Michael Neve, 'Public Views of Neurasthenia: Britain, 1880–1930', in Gijswijt-Hofstra and Porter (eds) *Cultures of Psychiatry*, p. 154.

25 Laura D. Hirshbein, *American Melancholy: Constructions of Depression in the Twentieth Century* (New Brunswick; London: Rutgers University Press, 2009), p. 17.

26 Lutz, 'Neurasthenia', p. 535.

27 Tom Lutz, *American Nervousness, 1903: An Anecdotal History* (Ithaca: Cornell University Press, 1991), p. 290.

28 Serge Doublet, *The Stress Myth* (Chesterfield, MO: Science & Humanities Press, 2000), p. 86.

29 *Ibid.*, pp. 162–3.

30 Patmore, *Truth*, p. 36.

31 Joan Busfield, *Men, Women and Madness: Understanding Gender and Mental Disorder* (Basingstoke: Macmillan, 1996), pp. 189–90.

32 Cooper and Dewe, *Stress*, pp. 117, 110–11.

33 Lawrence E. Hinkle, 'Stress and Disease: The Concept after 50 Years', *Social Science & Medicine* 25, 6 (1987): p. 561, https://doi.org/10.1016/0277-9536(87)90080-3.

34 Busfield, *Men, Women and Madness*, p. 190.

35 Cooper and Dewe, *Stress*, p. 112.

36 Russell Viner, 'Putting Stress in Life: Hans Selye and the Making of Stress Theory', *Social Studies of Science* 29, 3 (1999): p. 400, https://doi.org/10.1177/030631299029003003.

37 *Ibid.*, pp. 402–6; Jackson, *Age of Stress*, p. 168.

38 Busfield, *Men, Women and Madness*, p. 190.

39 David Wainwright and Michael Calnan, *Work Stress: The Making of a Modern Epidemic* (Buckingham: Open University Press, 2002), p. 44.

40 Dana Becker, *The Myth of Empowerment: Women and the Therapeutic Culture in America* (New York; London: New York University Press, 2005), p. 61.

41 Kristian Pollock, 'On the Nature of Social Stress: Production of a Modern Mythology', *Social Science & Medicine* 26, 3 (1988): p. 387, https://doi.org/10.1016/0277-9536(88)90404-2.

42 Ethan Watters, *Crazy Like Us: The Globalization of the American Psyche* (New York; London: Free Press, 2010), p. 6.

43 Doublet, *Stress Myth*, p. 78.

44 Hirshbein, *American Melancholy*, p. 17.

45 Viner, 'Putting Stress in Life', p. 391.

46 Robert A. Nye, 'The Evolution of the Concept of Medicalization in the Late Twentieth Century', *Journal of the History of the Behavioral Sciences* 39, 2 (2003): p. 124, https://doi.org/10.1002/jhbs.10108.

47 See for example, Elaine Showalter, *The Female Malady: Women, Madness, and English Culture, 1830–1980* (New York: Pantheon, 1985), p. 249; Busfield, *Men, Women and Madness*, p. 239.

48 Joan Busfield, 'Mental Illness', in Roger Cooter and John V. Pickstone (eds) *Companion to Medicine in the Twentieth Century* (London: Routledge, 2003), p. 640.

49 Roy Porter, *Madness: A Brief History* (Oxford: Oxford University Press, 2002), p. 214.

50 Edward Shorter, *A History of Psychiatry: From the Era of the Asylum to the Age of Prozac* (New York; Chichester: John Wiley & Sons, 1997), p. 178; Porter, *Madness*, p. 208.

51 Frank Füredi, *Therapy Culture: Cultivating Vulnerability in an Uncertain Age* (London; New York: Routledge, 2004), p. 98.

52 Nikolas Rose, *Governing the Soul: The Shaping of the Private Self* (London: Free Association, 1999), p. 125.

53 *Ibid.*, pp. 1–3.

54 Harold Perkin, *The Rise of Professional Society: England since 1880* (London; New York: Routledge, 1993), p. 418.

55 Füredi, *Therapy Culture*, 98; Avner Offer, *The Challenge of Affluence* (Oxford: Oxford University Press, 2006), p. 354; Wainwright and Calnan, *Work Stress*, p. 159.

56 Andrew Garrison, 'Restoring the Human in Humanistic Psychology', *Journal of Humanistic Psychology* 41, 4 (2001): p. 93.

57 Barbara Ehrenreich and Deirdre English, *For Her Own Good: 150 Years of the Experts' Advice to Women* (Garden City, NY: Anchor Press, 1978), p. 271.

58 Füredi, *Therapy Culture*, pp. 99, 106–7.

59 *Ibid.*, pp. 100–1; Wainwright and Calnan, *Work Stress*, p. 26.

60 Thomson, *Psychological Subjects*, p. 267; Füredi, *Therapy Culture*, p. 106; Rose, *Governing the Soul*, p. 258.

61 Mark S. Micale, 'The Psychiatric Body', in Cooter and Pickstone (eds) *Companion to Medicine*, p. 332; David Healy, *Let Them Eat Prozac* (New York; London: New York University Press, 2004), p. 264.

62 *Ibid.*

63 Füredi, *Therapy Culture*, p. 100; Rose, *Governing the Soul*, p. 125; Adrian Bingham, 'The "K-Bomb": Social Surveys, the Popular Press, and British Sexual Culture in the 1940s and 1950s', *The Journal of British Studies* 50, 1 (2011): p. 165; David Smail, *The Nature of Unhappiness* (London: Robinson, 2001), p. 23.

64 Nancy M. Theriot, 'Negotiating Illness: Doctors, Patients, and Families in the Nineteenth Century', *Journal of the History of the Behavioral Sciences* 37, 4 (2001): pp. 351–2, https://doi.org/10.1002/jhbs.1065.

65 Shorter, *History of Psychiatry*, p. 116.

66 Porter, *Madness*, p. 217; Janet Oppenheim, '*Shattered Nerves': Doctors, Patients, and Depression in Victorian England* (New York; Oxford: Oxford University Press, 1991), p. 15.

67 Tim Newton, Jocelyn Handy and Stephen Fineman, *Managing Stress: Emotion and Power at Work* (London; Thousand Oaks: Sage Publications, 1995), p. 2.

68 Nikolas Rose, 'Beyond Medicalisation', *The Lancet* 369, February 24 (2007): p. 700.

69 Healy, *Prozac*, p. 9; Ray Moynihan et al., 'Selling Sickness: The Pharmaceutical Industry and Disease Mongering', *BMJ* 324, 7342 (13 April 2002): p. 886, https://doi.org/10.1136/bmj.324.7342.886.

70 Christopher M. Callahan and German Elias Berrios, *Reinventing Depression: A History of the Treatment of Depression in Primary Care, 1940–2004* (Oxford: Oxford University Press, 2005), pp. 3, 30.

71 In Dean Rapp, 'The Reception of Freud by the British Press: General Interest and Literary Magazines, 1920–1925', *Journal of the History of the Behavioral Sciences* 24, 2 (1 April 1988): p. 193, https://doi.org/10.1002/1520-6696(198804)24:2<191::AID-JHBS2300240206>3.0.CO;2-X.

72 Thomson, *Psychological Subjects*, pp. 51–2.

73 Graham Richards, 'Britain on the Couch: The Popularization of Psychoanalysis in Britain 1918–1940', *Science in Context* 13, 2 (2000): p. 184, https://doi.org/10.1017/S0269889700003793; Thomson, *Psychological Subjects*, p. 209.

74 Barham, *Forgotten Lunatics*, p. 5; Thomson, *Psychological Subjects*, p. 185; Tracey Loughran, 'Shell-Shock and Psychological Medicine in First World War Britain', *Social History of Medicine* 22, 1 (April 2009): p. 91, https://doi.org/10.1093/shm/hkn093.

75 Thomson, *Psychological Subjects*, p. 34.

76 *Ibid.*, pp. 50–1.

77 Mathew Thomson, 'The Psychological Body', in Cooter and Pickstone (eds) *Companion to Medicine*, p. 295.

78 Joan Busfield, 'Class and Gender in Twentieth-Century British Psychiatry: Shell-Shock and Psychopathic Disorder', *Clio Medica / The Wellcome Series in the History of Medicine* 73 (2004): p. 303.

79 Jackson, *Age of Stress*, pp. 19, 191–3.

80 Garrison, 'Humanistic Psychology', p. 93.

81 Jackson, *Age of Stress*, p. 19.

82 Melling, 'Labouring Stress', p. 162.

83 Rose, *Governing the Soul*, p. 175.

84 Such as Füredi's *Therapy Culture*.

85 Eve Kosofsky Sedgwick, 'Epidemics of the Will', in Eve Kosofsky Sedgwick (ed.) *Tendencies* (London: Routledge, 1994), pp. 132–3; Mariana Valverde, *Diseases of the Will: Alcohol and the Dilemmas of Freedom* (Cambridge: Cambridge University Press, 1998), pp. 24–5.

86 Rose, *Governing the Soul*, p. 267.

87 *Ibid.*, p. 219.

88 Ehrenreich and English, *For Her Own Good*, pp. 268–9.

89 Richard Layard, *Happiness: Lessons from a New Science* (London: Penguin Group, 2005), p. 3; Offer, *Affluence*, p. 3; Oliver James, *Britain on the Couch* (London: Century, 1997), p. x.

90 Layard, *Happiness*, pp. 88–9.

91 Offer, *Affluence*, pp. 357–65.

92 Viner, 'Putting Stress in Life', p. 391.

93 Langhamer, '"Who the Hell Are Ordinary People?"', pp. 4, 7.

94 Highmore, *Everyday Life*, p. 7.

95 Selina Todd, 'Class, Experience and Britain's Twentieth Century', *Social History* 39, 4 (2014): p. 501, https://doi.org/10.1080/03071022.2014.983680. David Bloome, Dorothy Sheridan and Brian Street, 'Reading Mass Observation Writing: Theoretical and Methodological Issues in Researching in the Mass Observation Archive', *Mass Observation Archive Occasional Paper Series*, 1 (1996): p. 14.

96 Abrams and Brown, *Everyday Life in Scotland*, p. 1.

97 *Ibid.*, p. 3.

98 Alf Ludtke, 'What Is the History of Everyday Life and Who Are Its Practitioners?', in *The History of Everyday Life: Reconstructing Historical Experiences and Ways of Life*, trans. William Templer (Princeton, NJ: Princeton University Press, 1995), p. 3.

99 Roy Porter, 'The Patient's View: Doing Medical History From Below', *Theory and Society* 14, 2 (1985): pp. 175–98.

100 Flurin Condrau, 'The Patient's View Meets the Clinical Gaze', *Social History of Medicine* 20, 3 (2007): p. 529.

101 Michael Roper, 'Slipping Out of View: Subjectivity and Emotion in Gender History', *History Workshop Journal* 59, 1 (1 January 2005): p. 62, https://doi.org/10.1093/hwj/dbi006; Maria Tamboukou, 'Writing Genealogies: An Exploration of Foucault's Strategies for Doing Research', *Discourse: Studies in the Cultural Politics of Education* 20, 2 (1999): p. 202, https://doi.org/10.1080/0159630990200202.

102 Todd, 'Class, Experience and Britain's Twentieth Century', pp. 493–4.

103 For more on the history of MO see: James Hinton, *The Mass Observers: A History, 1937–1949* (Oxford: Oxford University Press, 2013); Nick Hubble, *Mass Observation and Everyday Life: Culture, History, Theory* (Basingstoke: Palgrave Macmillan, 2006); Tom Jeffrey, *Mass Observation: A Short History* (Brighton: MOA, 1999); Penny Summerfield, 'Mass Observation: Social Research or Social Movement', *Journal of Contemporary History* 20, 3 (1985).

104 Claire Langhamer, *The English in Love: The Intimate Story of an Emotional Revolution* (Oxford: Oxford University Press, 2013), p. xvi. For a thorough discussion of methodological concerns about the MOA and MOP, see Annebella Pollen, 'Research Methodology in Mass Observation Past and Present: "Scientifically, about as Valuable as a Chimpanzee's Tea Party at the Zoo"?', *History Workshop Journal*, 75 (Spring 2013), https://doi.org/10.1093/hwj/dbs040.

105 Hubble, *Mass Observation and Everyday Life*, p. 8.

106 Bloome, Sheridan and Street, 'Reading Mass Observation', pp. 10–11.

107 Pollen, 'Research Methodology', p. 11.

108 Jeff Mills, Millennium Memory Bank Collection, 12 September 1998, C900/05537, British Library Sound Archive © BBC.

109 See for example Joanna Bornat, Parvati Raghuram and Leroi Henry, 'Revisiting the Archives: A Case Study from the History of Geriatric Medicine', *Sociological Research Online* 17, 2 (2012), www.socresonline.org.uk/17/2/1.html; Jo Haynes and Demelza Jones, 'A Tale of Two Analyses: The Use of Archived Qualitative Data', *Sociological Research Online* 17, 2 (2012): p. 1.

110 Joanna Bornat, 'A Second Take: Revisiting Interviews with a Different Purpose', *Oral History* 31, 1 (2003): p. 49, https://doi.org/10.2307/40179735.

111 April Gallwey, 'The Rewards of Using Archival Oral Histories in Research: The Case of the Millennium Memory Bank', *Oral History* 41, 1 (2013): p. 38.

112 Rob Perks, 'The Century Speaks: A Public History Partnership', *Oral History* 29, 2 (2001): pp. 95, 97, https://doi.org/10.2307/40179712.

113 Gallwey, 'Archival Oral Histories', p. 47.

114 Bingham, *Family Newspapers?* pp. 2–3.

115 Elizabeth Siegel Watkins, 'Stress and the American Vernacular', in Cantor and Ramsden (eds) *Stress, Shock, and Adaptation*, p. 50.

116 For example: Oppenheim, *'Shattered Nerves'*; Edward Shorter, *How Everyone Became Depressed: The Rise and Fall of the Nervous Breakdown* (Oxford: Oxford University Press, 2013); Haggett, *Male Psychological Disorders*.

117   Watkins, 'American Vernacular', p. 50.
118   Viner, 'Putting Stress in Life', p. 391.
119   Jackson, *Age of Stress*, pp. 141–80.
120   Richard Asher, *Nerves Explained: A Straightforward Guide to Nervous Illnesses* (London: Faber and Faber, 1957), p. 19.
121   For example, Haggett, *Desperate Housewives*.

1

Nerves and the nervous: self-help books in the early decades of the twentieth century

Britain in the early twentieth century was a stressful place to live. According to Dr Edwin Hopewell Ash, writing a book for the nervous in 1928, 'everything is being speeded up more and more'. Not only were many people still coming to terms with the psychological after-effects of the First World War, but they were 'working at full pressure to meet present conditions, travelling hundreds of miles in a week-end, dancing into the early hours of the morning'. Adding to this already hectic life were news services bringing the 'most interesting, varied and exciting events' from all over the world almost as soon as they occurred. If that were not enough, there were also the marvels of wireless and the 'excitements of flying'. The speed and sophistication of such modernity were all very well, noted Ash, but unfortunately, it put a strain on the nerves that urgently needed attention.[1]

Ash was a doctor specialising in nervous diseases, who worked in several London hospitals and through a series of popular works, was one of several writers aiming to help the general population deal with such challenges in the early decades of the twentieth century.[2] Like him, many were doctors keen to offer advice for the nervous in easily understood lay terms. Although this sort of book was by no means new – building on a rich tradition of medical self-help books – a boom in psychological advice books at the beginning of the century reflected the growing interest in popular psychology and the increasing market for 'self-help' publications, although publishers did not yet recognise or categorise such works thus. Self-help books allowed the reader to negotiate meaning for their experiences without engaging with formal medical diagnoses which might legitimise or dismiss their worries, both of which could be troubling. They ensured privacy and, not

surprisingly, were underpinned by an assumption of reader agency
and self-sufficiency. They framed the nervous reader as intelligent
enough to recognise the need for help, but sufficiently capable to learn
about, understand and treat their condition themselves.

The early century was notable for a growing fascination with the
psyche reflected in enthusiasm for occultism and spiritualism, as well
as mental training systems such as Pelmanism, and saw a boom in
books of psychological guidance.[3] Increased levels of literacy, expansion
of mass media and a growing drive for self-improvement meant that
the issues and concerns that might previously have been largely limited
to the domain of politicians and professionals, became much more
available to a popular audience.[4] Public interest in psychology was
fuelled by debates over shell shock and its treatment, and in many
cases by the struggle to obtain pensions. Ultimately 120,000 veterans
of the First World War were given pensions for psychiatric disability,
more than a quarter of them still being paid in 1937.[5] Although mental
illness carried a considerable stigma, and the treatment of shell-shocked
veterans was heavily bounded by class assumptions, their presence in
the general population ensured an increased awareness of the potential
frailties of the psyche among the lay population as well as the institutions
of medicine and government.[6] This was reflected in the appearance
of afflicted veterans in popular culture such as Dorothy L. Sayer's
aristocratic sleuth, Lord Peter Wimsey, one of whose suspects in the
1928 novel *The Unpleasantness at the Bellona Club* is a fellow shell
shock sufferer.[7]

The psychological scars of the First World War were accompanied
by a loss of faith and confidence in the world that was reinforced by
the economic vagaries of the interwar period.[8] The intermittent
unemployment of the Depression of the 1930s created insecurity,
anxiety, humiliation and loss of self-esteem in the men affected and
permeated the lives of their families. According to contemporary
research this provided fertile ground for mental instability and neurasthenia, which in turn fed into concerns, particularly in the 1930s,
that such mind states could be contagious, an idea that was increasingly
current in popular culture and news reporting, apparently demonstrated
by the spread of fascism in Europe.[9] This contributed to a widespread
culture of decline and crisis that for Richard Overy created an 'undif-
ferentiated sense of malaise'.[10] In many cases those turning to self-help

books were undoubtedly looking for ways to manage this feeling and deal with their own nervous suffering or that of someone close to them, whether caused by the war or wider issues.

Such hunger for psychological knowledge owed less to Freud and psychoanalysis and more to an eclectic British interpretation of such ideas based on a psychology of self-improvement rather than the breaking down of the self required by psychoanalysis.[11] At the same time, increasing secularism and the development of mass marketing and new opportunities for leisure offered what Thomson has called 'commodity solutions' to constructions of health and treatments for illness so that by the late 1930s popular psychology was embraced in newspaper advice columns, correspondence courses, psychology clubs and a range of self-help books. Their content tended to reflect a psychology that drew on lingering Victorian values of self-control and moral management as well as the new possibilities of upward mobility through self-improvement.[12]

Drawing on a sample of self-help books, published between 1907 and the outbreak of the Second World War, this chapter examines popular explanations and treatments for nervous conditions as well as the wide range of symptoms constituting those ailments. These books were selected specifically because they were intended for a lay readership, albeit a mostly middle-class, educated one. They deployed the concepts and terminology more likely to be accessible and taken up by the ordinary reader, as opposed to more medical and technical texts designed for a specialist audience, although the latter might also be among their readership.[13] The variety of symptoms discussed by self-help authors indicated just how broad the parameters of popular conceptions of nerves and nervousness were for authors and sufferers alike. Popular understanding of nerves also revealed the privileging of certain explanations, symptoms and treatments as well as the contemporary gender and class assumptions that informed interpretations of causality and proposed remedies. Self-help books reveal how contemporary notions of health and well-being, stoicism and personal responsibility underpinned the way nervous suffering was understood. They highlight concepts such as self-responsibility, personal agency and the privileging of physical symptoms. Such ideas continued to inform popular understanding of nerves and ultimately stress for much of the century.

Self-help books

Ash's concerns about the effects of modern life on Britain's population were by no means new. Indeed the diagnosis of neurasthenia in the nineteenth century had been based on similar ideas about the effects of too much work, speed and mental effort.[14] Hence, although the idea was not a new one, the turn towards nerves and away from neurasthenia as a diagnosis in the early twentieth century reflected changes in the ways in which professional medicine, personal experience and popular culture were constructing the language of psychological ill-health at the time.[15] The pernicious effects of modernity on the human psyche were already evident in earlier self-help titles such as *Worry: The Disease of the Age* and *Why Worry?* published in 1907 and 1908, respectively, and Ash himself had already published several volumes about nerves, including *Nerves and the Nervous* in 1911 and *The Problem of Nervous Breakdown* in 1919.[16] Ideas about the dangers of advancing civilisation had a long history and similar concerns continued to be repeated regularly throughout the twentieth century, with frequent suggestions that contemporary life was somehow uniquely challenging, and the pace of change particularly rapid.[17] Overy contends that the interwar period was particularly prey to this anxiety about civilisation, partly because the horrors of the recent war had proven its fragility but also because of new ideas drawn from Freudian thinking that implied that civilisation was but a thin veneer hiding man's inner demons.[18] Such notions threatened the social order and fuelled concerns about the pace of change and its effects on sexual morality, class, race and mental health. These anxieties undoubtedly drove the increased enthusiasm of the public for help in understanding, managing and treating their troubled nerves.

Most self-help authors were either doctors or psychiatrists and, except for Flora Klickmann who was a journalist and Josephine A. Jackson who was a psychiatrist, the authors discussed in this chapter were all men. This undoubtedly reflected the limited number of women in relevant professions who were able and willing to publish a self-help book, at the time. Many of the authors drew explicitly on their experience with patients, often using examples of conversations with them and adopting the vernacular language of nerves. It is perhaps for this reason that few of them referred to cutting-edge developments in

scientific, medical or psychiatric research, although one or two mentioned the work of Walter Cannon in the period and the idea of the
'flight or fight' response.[19] They offered a straightforward approach to
dealing with psychological suffering that also largely eschewed the
complexities of psychoanalysis, and addressed the kind of questions
and assumptions that the 'average' reader looking for help with a problem
might have. This reflected the unfavourable reception of psychoanalytic
ideas, particularly Freud's sexual theories, among many doctors and
lay people, as well as the very practical need for any suggested remedies
to be accessible to, and achievable by, readers themselves.[20] Those
seeking help in a book were probably not willing or financially able to
discuss their mental health difficulties with a professional. This
pragmatic approach mirrored the approach of GPs, as the British Medical
Association (BMA) found in the late 1920s when it carried out research
into the implications of psychoanalytic ideas for general practice. Most
GPs took a practical approach and treated mild neurosis with encouragement, tonics, holidays and sedatives.[21] Self-help books followed a
similar model.

This was one area where British self-help books differed from their
American counterparts, which were nevertheless influential in the
British market. In the USA there had long been a flourishing market
in self-help books. Initially grounded in religion and the development
of good character and sound ethical beliefs, underpinned by self-control
and the harnessing of inner spiritual energy, by the beginning of the
twentieth century these books were increasingly focused on broader
ideas of human potential coming from psychology and incorporating
all aspects of living.[22] During the interwar period, partly as a response
to the economic and social upheavals resulting from war and the
Depression and partly to the growth of psychotherapy, they increasingly focused on helping the reader cope with the strain of modern
life.[23] Among the most prolific US authors was Walter B. Pitkin, a
university professor whose much-imitated works included *Life Begins
at Forty*, and *More Power to You: A Working Technique for Making the
Most of Human Energy*.[24] Similarly, Dale Carnegie's *How to Win Friends
and Influence People* was effectively a how-to guide to success, and
certainly worked for its author, selling 759,000 hardback copies on
publication in 1937 and more than 30 million copies worldwide over
the rest of the century.[25] Such books represented the emergence of

a western cultural phenomenon informed less by Christianity and more by the demands of industrial organisation and new economic markets. Whatever the case, the success of self-help books in the USA undoubtedly influenced British publishers and changes to the publishing industry in the early century resulting from new transatlantic agreements led to an increase in sales of American titles in Britain so that a significant number of US self-help books were successfully produced in British editions.[26]

While some of the American books offered a more psychoanalytical product, their appeal lay in their often more vernacular tone and use of humour, seen in book and chapter titles such as *Be Glad You're Neurotic* and *Even Dogs Get Neurotic.*[27] These books and their British equivalents were a staple of many of the major publishing houses such as George Allen & Unwin in Britain and McGraw Hill in the USA, and were also the focus of more specialist publishers such as William Rider & Son, and Mills & Boon. For many publishers, the titles in their educational lists (a likely category for such books) provided the solid sales which supported riskier literary ventures.[28] Although in the early century the readership of self-help books was restricted to those who were literate and had access to books, some were produced as simple leaflets of a few dozen pages on poor-quality paper, implying their reach could extend to the working as well as middle classes, and access expanded considerably as the century progressed, aided by libraries and the popularisation of cheap paperbacks in the 1930s.[29]

Because such books were not part of a specific genre of publishing it is difficult to quantify their popularity based on sales, as they were subsumed within various other categories such as education or even philosophy, in records such as *The Bookseller.*[30] However, the frequency of reprints and the longevity of some titles such as *Nerves in Disorder,* published in 1903 and then reprinted in 1918 and 1927, or *You Must Relax: A Practical Method of Reducing the Strains of Modern Living,* which was first released in 1934 and was still being reprinted in its fifth, revised and enlarged edition in 1980, indicates a significant level of popularity.[31] Publishers would have been unlikely to reprint without a recognised demand. There were evidently people who wished to seek solutions to their nervous suffering in books rather than consulting their GP. This may have been to avoid the expense of a medical consultation, to preserve their privacy or to enable them to care for someone else. The last is certainly suggested by the range of titles published after the First World War, surely aimed at veterans and their families, though this was only very occasionally acknowledged by authors, few of whom addressed the effects of the war directly.[32] This was possibly because the problems of the shell shocked could not realistically be dealt with in a self-help book or perhaps to ensure as wide a readership as possible. Ash and William Loosmore, of Glasgow University, both referred to the potential for nervous problems to arise as an after-effect of the strain of war, and this perhaps reflects the perceived purview of their books: they were not intended to address the potentially extreme psychological damage of shell shock but might reasonably be used as a source of help for those with more general nervous strain.[33]

Most authors aimed to address a lay readership in language that they could understand: Ash explains in the preface to *Nerves and the Nervous* in 1911 that his book was written in 'non-technical language, and with a view to the instruction of the lay-reader'.[34] Stated motivations for writing self-help books revealed contemporary concerns and changing social needs. Dougall MacDougall King, whose brother was the Canadian prime minister, published *Nerves and Personal Power* in 1923, and was concerned to ensure that social workers, religious teachers and the legal professions gained a wider knowledge of nervousness, while Alfred Schofield, a Harley Street physician, in his 1927 work wanted to dispel ignorance about nerve diseases, which many regarded 'as either shams or frauds'.[35] Both authors were undoubtedly reflecting the difficulties thrown up by shell shock cases from the war and the range of professionals likely to be called on for help. Contemporary with them, Jackson hoped to improve psychiatric knowledge among GPs, presumably for much the same reasons.[36] Several authors wrote from the perspective of being a sufferer of nervous conditions themselves, which made them evangelical about their own supposed cure but also implied a certain empathy with the reader. Such admissions were also claims to authenticity based not on expertise, but on experience, which might carry more weight with readers suspicious of psychiatry. For example, William Kendall recounted in the early 1930s that his book, *The Conquest of Nerves*, was 'an attempt to explain a way of overcoming "nerves" which the writer has worked out with help from many sources'. He hoped to make the method more widely known because it had 'proved successful in freeing the writer himself and others from bondage to morbid fear and depression'.[37] Such admissions, blurring the line between professional and patient, while undoubtedly aimed at reassuring and convincing the reader, also displayed a marked lack of the usual shame associated with mental health problems, and again can be seen as a legacy of the increased awareness of psychological problems among the British public resulting from the First World War. They also suggest that some of the association of nervous conditions with higher social status, originally seen in understandings of neurasthenia in the nineteenth century, still lingered. Louis Bisch, an American psychiatrist writing in the 1930s, certainly positioned the idea of neuroticism as something which set the sufferer apart, arguing that 'to be normal is nothing to brag about!' and the title of his book, *Be Glad You're Neurotic*, underlined his stance.[38]

The titles of self-help books reveal much about the ways that nerves and nervousness were conceptualised and marketed through language. These popular terms lacked the precision of medical diagnoses, and for that reason were useful in encompassing a vast array of experiences from the mild to the severe. They were also considerably less threatening than the formal psychiatric labels available and allowed for individual interpretation that could emphasise or minimise symptoms. This made them useful to a variety of readers and might account for the longevity not just of some of the books, but also the popular terminology that they employed. Book titles reflected commercial concerns and authorial preferences but commonly fell into four categories: instructive, combative, familiar and descriptive. They reflected contemporary concerns. Among the many instructive titles, *Mending Your Nerves* and *How to Train Your Nerves* both implied firstly that nerves could be broken, which was consistent with the interwar conceptualisation of shell-shocked veterans, and secondly that they could be trained, which was consonant with the emerging enthusiasm for health, hygiene and physical fitness.[39] Combative titles such as *The Conquest of Nerves* or *Outwitting our Nerves* implied an understanding of nervous disorders as potentially overwhelming, as something which needed to be 'outwitted' or 'safeguarded' against and which required vigilance and self-control.[40] Underlying this was the age-old fear of lunacy and of unknown forces within which might overwhelm the individual, and the popularisation of ideas about the Freudian unconscious in the early part of the century no doubt reinforced this.[41] Such a framework also included ideas about mental degeneracy, weakness of character, heredity and personality which emphasised how the individual contained within him- or herself both the seeds of their own condition and the agency to guard or fight against it. By contrast, titles using familiar language attempted to downplay the fearfulness of mental distress by treating it dismissively, as in *Those Nerves*, or comfortingly, such as *Making Friends with our Nerves*.[42] Descriptive titles were largely consistent across the period and despite the apparent gender specificity of some titles, such as *Nerves and the Man*, were usually aimed at both men and women, although the approach and suggested treatments within were often gendered.[43]

During the early decades of the twentieth century, self-help books constituted one of the informal means of support and education to which people turned when looking for help with their troubles.[44] For many, those troubles seemed rife. The impact of the First World War and anxieties about the possibility of another, coupled with economic turbulence and social change, gave the public an appetite for knowledge about and the vocabulary with which to express such worries.[45] The idea of psychological suffering became normalised as part of modern life, and so, arguably, seeking help to deal with it also became normalised, although it still needed to be managed with discretion. There were undoubtedly many reasons why people chose to buy or borrow a book rather than consulting a doctor. Certainly there was a high level of stigma still attached to mental illness, and the 'haunting dread of insanity' still created a powerful disincentive for admitting concern about the state of one's psyche.[46] Although half of the working population had access to panel doctors by the end of the interwar period, this excluded wives and children, and for many there was still a sense that consulting the doctor, held in awe as somewhere between a 'saint and a god', was only to be done in cases of life or death.[47] Visiting such paragons was therefore not done lightly, and while many doctors were kind, helpful and caring, there were also those whose attitude to the sort of symptoms that might present as 'nervousness' was summarily dismissive. On the other hand, the very action of consulting a doctor might create anxiety as it effectively legitimised symptoms which previously only the sufferer had known about. Whatever the case, self-help books offered an alternative which could reassure the reader that they were not going mad and offer practical suggestions for actions they could take themselves to address their problem. They were also a fundamental part of a burgeoning popular psychological culture that emphasised personal agency and the potential of self-development and thus provided their readers with a sense of taking control which, in itself, might be sufficient to help them deal with their troubles.

Symptoms

Descriptions of symptoms in self-help books enabled readers to compare their own experiences and, the authors hoped, recognise them and learn how to deal with them. Symptoms were often divided between the physical, the behavioural and the mental or psychological, with a distinct emphasis on the first in the early part of the century, reflecting the dominance of somatic explanations of illness. This was because in popular understanding a physical symptom must have a physical cause, and therefore was a distinct proof against any hint of lunacy. An individual would be much more likely to admit to a physical symptom, even if it was effectively a proxy for something more psychological. Clearly, self-help authors could not address the extreme conditions of psychosis and trauma, so by their very nature the identification of symptoms was grounded in the everyday and related to experiences which were frequent, ongoing and often commonplace. While this undoubtedly helped to address the concerns of the reader, it also inevitably pathologised many of the previously mundane experiences of daily life and contributed to a growing medicalisation of everyday existence in the early decades of the twentieth century.

Fatigue was the classic symptom of neurasthenics in the nineteenth century and it appeared frequently, along with associated insomnia, in many self-help books; for example in his 1920 book *Nerves and the Man*, Loosmore talked of the 'upsetting of sleep habits', while Milton Powell, a 'Diet Specialist and Nature Cure Practitioner', identified symptoms of 'intense fatigue'.[48] Authors might differ considerably on other symptoms, but problems with sleep and resultant tiredness were consistent across the period. Arguably fatigue could result from a multiplicity of causes, many of them physical and with nothing at all to do with nerves or stress. However, its frequency of appearance serves to illustrate the breadth of reader experiences which self-help authors were trying to address, and the mutability of the whole concept. For in practice there would be few readers who could not admit to suffering fatigue at some point in their lives.

Another frequently mentioned symptom was digestive problems, often synonymous with constipation or ulcers. The link between emotional strain and digestive health was by no means new, but as Hayward and Jones have established, its emergence in very particular forms, such as 'busman's stomach' in the 1930s and the epidemic of dyspepsia during the Second World War, was often a cultural phenomenon resulting from quite specific contemporary popular health concerns, and political and social circumstances.[49] Nevertheless, authors recognised the prevalence of such physical symptoms – although as one tactfully put it, the sufferer's 'tired feeling' might well be due to 'inadequate intestinal elimination' while another suggested that the 'strange "sensations" that always accompany nerve-weakness' were often due to 'nothing more romantic than flatulence!'[50] Powell proposed that nerves might be 'poisoned' by too much processed food and 'starved' from insufficient vegetables, while others reported loss of appetite as a symptom.[51] Headaches were also prevalent, Loosmore reporting that patients complained of their head feeling like it was 'being pressed', while other physical symptoms included trembling limbs, restlessness, faintness, giddiness, nausea and 'a wobbly feeling at the heart'.[52] Such physical symptoms were of great import to sufferers in proving that they were not imagining their sufferings: the bodily pain or malfunction was proof of a physical problem. Although many of the self-help authors framed nervous disorders as psychological rather than physical in cause, their tacit acknowledgement of readers' need to conceptualise their problems physically offered a means of countering accusations that the reader's problem was all in the mind or the result of hypochondria, and reinforced the idea that it could be tackled practically.

More psychological symptoms included irritability and craving for excitement, depression, low self-confidence, timidity and a 'recurring sense of vague and indefinable fears'.[53] Some of them were the result of physical symptoms, with Ash explaining that 'Exhaustion and headache lasting for some time cannot fail to produce very great depression', while Powell also attributed depression to 'nerve exhaustion' and 'an unstable nervous system'.[54] Resulting behavioural symptoms described by authors included dislike of meeting strangers, 'fear to cross the road, of open or enclosed spaces, fear of financial collapse of travelling by train or attending theatres.'[55] These were likely to make the sufferer 'unhappy and inefficient in his work' as well as 'self-conscious and oversensitive'.[56] Other signs of nervous breakdown included loss of memory and introspection where 'the mind is so occupied with itself that interest in outside and natural things is almost absent'.[57] Such introspection might lead to 'dreads, fancies, fixed ideas, morbid thoughts, suspicions', and include 'dread of losing reason'.[58] Thus many authors went to great lengths to assure readers that suffering from nerves was not the first step to madness, the anonymous author of *From Terror to Triumph* explaining that 'Many neurasthenics think that they are going insane. Do you? Well, that is your guarantee that you won't. No man went mad who *thought* he would.'[59]

Such symptoms were perhaps not so surprising in a period in which the challenges of everyday life were played out against a backdrop of apparent decline, crisis, pessimism and dismay, as Overy has argued.[60] During the 1920s unemployment remained at or above one million of the insured population and increased to three million after the Wall Street crash in 1929. In such circumstances, only the very rich were truly free from the fear of unemployment and potential destitution, and the intermittent pattern of employment experienced by many men created an ongoing insecurity and anxiety for them and their families for years.[61] Worries about unemployment only began to be alleviated in the late 1930s, but by then the international situation and fears of the inevitability of another war, which had been a growing part of popular discourse since the early 1930s, meant that people's minds were increasingly troubled by fear of impending conflict and the memories this brought back of the last war.[62] In such circumstances, it was perhaps inevitable that many experienced 'vague and indefinable fears' and sought a means to alleviate them.[63]

Any individual who felt they were suffering from a nervous condition and who picked up a self-help book as remedy was almost certain to find symptoms described with which they could identify. Whether it was vague fears, digestive issues, timidity or spending too much time dwelling on their problems, in practice most self-help authors offered sufficient variety of symptoms to enable readers to conclude that the book could offer some help for their specific case. While undoubtedly such variety was partly offered in good faith, it also meant that the books would be relevant to as many readers as possible, and thus more marketable. What this meant in turn was that many everyday, as well as pathological, experiences could fall within the popular nervous remit.

Causes

The wide variety of causes suggested in these books also appealed to a range of different reader experiences and included the speed of modern life, brain work, gender roles, heredity and overindulgence in food, exciting popular entertainments and even sex. As such, causation was both complex and fluid and allowed readers to interpret their own experiences in a variety of ways, according to what made sense and was acceptable to them and others. The stated causes reflected contemporary society and assumptions about class and gender, particularly in relation to status, occupation and role. They also highlighted the role of personal choice and responsibility for lifestyle, which effectively laid the blame for some nervous suffering at the feet of the reader, presenting authors with a challenge in explaining this without alienating their audience. Several explanations, such as the strains of modern life and work, would have considerable longevity, continuing to contribute to the late twentieth-century popular discourse of stress.

Ash's comments at the beginning of this chapter are typical of many writers who saw the most obvious cause of nervous conditions as the current state of modern life. The First World War had demonstrated the horrifying potential of new technologies with death and destruction on an unprecedented scale, and this undoubtedly affected how people perceived notions of progress and modernity. According to Schofield, modern life was creating nervous sufferers all over the world, but especially in France, England and the USA, which he deemed to be the most advanced nations, and his comments reflected contemporary eugenic concerns about the decline of modern populations.[64] Official reports in the early 1920s suggested a worryingly high level of unfit or defective individuals in the British population, including the finding that of two-and-a-half million men examined in the last year of the war, only three in nine were fit, the rest being infirm, chronic invalids or only capable of limited work.[65] Such pronouncements fuelled a sense of panic about the state of the nation and underpinned a preoccupation with improving the race reflected in the activities of the eugenic movement in Britain.[66] This was particularly focused on halting national degeneration linked to concerns about maintenance of the Empire, coupled with the hope that application of scientific principles could lead to human progress. Although these ideas dated back to the late nineteenth century, they reached their high point of influence in the early twentieth century, in organisations such as the Eugenics Education Society and the founding of a chair of Eugenics at University College London, and eugenic ideas were reflected in many self-help books, particularly in linking the causes of nervous suffering to social status, heredity and the threats inherent in modern life for those constitutionally unsuited to it.[67]

Ash argued that part of the problem was 'the enormous stress of life under the conditions in which it is lived in the great cities of the world', situating the problem as a specifically urban one.[68] Significant was the traffic congestion, noise and bustle which increased the 'brain strain of trying to get about safely and across roads without mishap'.[69] In his 1911 book, he went so far as to identify 'Chauffeurs' Nerves' as a unique condition brought about by the 'undue strain' of 'controlling motor-vehicles', especially in the crowded traffic of London.[70] However, the category failed to appear in later works, presumably because by then motor traffic had become a normal part of everyday life in cities, although the emergence of 'busman's stomach' in the 1930s evidently drew on similar concerns, and both conditions were notable for affecting working-class sufferers.[71] Its disappearance also reflected the fact that most self-help books were little concerned with the troubles of the working classes, tending to focus on their more likely middle-class audience.

Indeed, talk of chauffeurs reflected the social order of the Britain in which Ash and his readers lived: one of clear social distinctions and an often eugenic view of class differences. However, it was a society that was changing, and several authors, Ash among them, saw such changes as causes of nervous disorders. He wrote that 'money that a former generation saved thriftily is today spent like water by a vast pleasure-loving multitude that lives only for the present', while Schofield was concerned that pursuit of money occurred 'at the expense of the wear-and-tear of nerve'.[72] Ash's comments seem particularly critical of the opportunities for leisure becoming more accessible and affordable to the working classes, notably in the interwar period. In a similar vein, writing in the 1930s, Walter Wolfe, who was director of a Community Church Mental Hygiene Clinic, appeared critical of social mobility, explaining, 'Analyze an unhappy life and you will usually find that the unhappy man has either set his goal of security and satisfaction beyond the pale of human attainment, or beyond the bounds of social approval.'[73] Wolfe appeared to be implying that ambition and failure to know one's place could damage mental health.

The potential threat of social change, industrialisation, urbanisation and subsequent technological transformation was part of the repeating theme that contemporary life was damaging to the psyche, traceable back to the nineteenth century and earlier, and repeated throughout the twentieth century.[74] While it was certainly the case that many of the results of such changes were physically damaging, such as traffic and air pollution, what such a belief about modern life also suggested was a human response to a sense of powerlessness in the face of change. Arguably throughout the nineteenth and twentieth centuries each generation perceived the world to be changing more quickly and to be more challenging and potentially pernicious than the last. The success of self-help books in America, particularly in the 1930s, has been attributed to a perception that technical innovations had outstripped human ability, and self-help provided one solution to fitting and equipping humans to their new environment, which was vital to the success of American civilisation.[75] In practice, the majority of people, most of the time, had little influence or ability to affect the societal and economic changes around them, thus one response to sometimes bewildering or threatening change was to attribute the distress of such powerlessness to those very external factors themselves.

While concerns about the harmful effects of modern life were suggestive of certain attitudes towards class, the attribution of nervous conditions to overuse of the brain was undoubtedly illustrative of the powerful class determinants among many authors' explanations of causation. Brain work implied a problem of the educated and professional, invariably male and middle class, as Loosmore's identification of clergymen, politicians, lawyers and heads of business as sufferers illustrates.[76] This was a continuation of the neurasthenic tradition that overworking the brain was dangerous. As Ash explained, 'We begin to see how persistent work on the same lines, even if never amounting to painful stress, may so steadily fatigue the brain cells that their vitality is eventually impaired.'[77] In simple terms, working the brain too hard depleted nerve energy which in turn could lead to a range of symptoms and ultimately breakdown. Class distinctions were further emphasised by the explicit association of nervous conditions with superior status, some authors claiming famous historical figures as nerve sufferers, such as Alexander the Great, Caesar and Napoleon.[78] There was also the indication of a quid pro quo: the compensation for sufferers of nervous breakdown was that 'if they suffer much, they also enjoy much', presumably because of their greater sensitivity and refinement.[79] Bisch in the 1930s went so far as to state, 'I'm a neurotic myself and delighted.'[80] Whether such declarations were intended to create empathy with the reader or simply reflected authorial arrogance is difficult to judge, but the intention at the very least was to suggest that the reader was in good company. Nerves were clearly a product of a sensitivity which arose only in certain 'types', usually associated with favourable social or material standing.

Such 'types' might be prone to highlighting their sensitivity to gain attention, or to relieve boredom, and Ash commented that many doctors would be familiar with cases of women from wealthy families presenting with nervous disorders which were largely the result of them having 'nothing to do'.[81] Similarly, Bisch referred to the sense of importance that might accompany self-identification as nervous, and George Walton, a neurologist and fellow American, described 'the melancholy pleasures of playing the martyr'.[82] This issue highlights a critical concern about nervous conditions: how to judge whether someone was genuinely suffering or faking it for their own ends. The multiplicity of potential nervous symptoms allowed the sufferer or opportunist to co-opt their own meaning, which was difficult to challenge and could be played up or down as the situation demanded. It is notable that most suggestions in self-help books about the faking of illness or adoption of a patient identity related to the behaviour of the leisured and middle classes, reflecting the social identity of both authors and their potential readership.

This, in itself, reveals the almost wholesale absence of attention to working-class experience of nervous disorders. Only Ash in *Nerves and the Nervous* openly acknowledged that nervous disorders *did* cross class *and* gender boundaries, as he explained: 'Artisans, labourers, porters, women who probably never open a book or write a line, domestic servants and navvies are by no means free from such afflictions, and

I have some of the worst cases amongst patients of this class.' However, he attributed different causes which continued to deny working-class sufferers any claim on the cultural capital of brain work, suggesting that 'monotony of life, poor circumstances, and the innumerable worries associated therewith' were the causes of their suffering.[83] No doubt one reason that most authors did not address the nervous conditions of the working classes was that, as Ash alluded to, few were likely readers, having little access to books and even less time or money for them, although this was changing during the interwar period. Klickmann's 1925 book did address white-collar female workers 'in offices', reflecting the increasing numbers of women in clerical and shop work in the 1920s.[84] Her book, however, was exceptional not only in targeting a broader demographic but also in treating women's activities both inside and outside the home as work.

Many authors did not distinguish between male and female sufferers in their books; however, for those who did, it appeared that simply being a woman could be a cause of nervous suffering. This was certainly not a new idea, as Janet Oppenheim has argued; the idea of female health being undermined by inherent weakness is traceable back to Aristotle but became particularly noteworthy in the Victorian period, partly thanks to the ideas of evolutionary biology.[85] By the early twentieth century the idea was much less explicit, and in self-help books the cause of female nervous suffering was largely attributed to the roles that women performed. Thus, a lack of meaningful occupation on the one hand and too much emphasis on perfecting housework on the other could make women unwell. Walton commented on the dangers of becoming obsessive about cleaning where 'it gives one a "fit" to see a picture slightly off the level, and drives one "wild" to see a speck of dust', although as the women he and most of the other authors were describing were largely middle class and wealthy, they were not the ones actually doing the cleaning.[86] There was no discussion of the effects of a mistress going 'wild' about a speck of dust on the nerves of her housemaid. Talking about women living in suburbs and country towns, Ash claimed that 'the deadly monotony of life' caused the 'development of nervous troubles which seem to occur from sheer starvation of the higher mental faculties', a conclusion which was echoed in the diagnosis of 'suburban neurosis', as the next chapter will discuss, and which featured in post-war debates about the potentially atrophying confines of women's domestic lives as well as informing 'The Problem that has No Name' in Betty Friedan's groundbreaking 1960s work, *The Feminine Mystique*.[87]

The danger was apparent as soon as a female left education, according to Schofield. The abrupt cessation of a full daily timetable left girls with little more to do than arrange flowers for half an hour a day, which could have a marked effect on the nerves.[88] However, even if she weathered such tedium, married and set up her own home, a woman could expect further problems from motherhood. Klickmann argued that a mother could not 'close her desk at five o'clock, and get away from her business problems' as her responsibilities were 'ever with her, waking or sleeping'.[89] With some prescience she homed in on the core of the problem for women, their lack of agency and control of their own destiny, noting, 'Sometimes one sees a mother sacrificing all her own personal inclinations in order to give her children a good time; or a wife reduced to a colourless nonentity by a selfish dominating husband; or a daughter deprived of the ordinary pleasures and pursuits of young womanhood by the exacting demands of an invalid parent.'[90] She was unusual in also addressing the dual working roles of women, explaining that 'the girl, who is herself very likely tired out and strained with the bad air of a City office, to say nothing of her business responsibilities, is not in the mood to tackle household worries or work when she comes home'.[91] This issue of balancing full-time employment and domestic responsibilities would only really come to the fore during the Second World War, when concern over recruitment of women to war work and absenteeism among the workforce forced the government to acknowledge the challenges of the dual burden, although it would become a staple of debates about women's roles from then on, adding to the perceived causes of female stress in the late century.[92]

Balance was at the heart of another frequently cited source of nervous suffering: overindulgence. While overtaxing the brain could be problematic, so could too much fun. Loosmore cautioned his readers that 'many are the victims who sacrifice their nerve forces upon the altar of amusement and pleasure'.[93] Whether this involved 'the stress of a London season, with its endless round of dinners, theatres, balls and receptions' or even visiting friends and going to plays, many authors agreed that these were an 'obvious cause of nerve-exhaustion', although obviously only to those classes that could afford them.[94] The digestive system was again a focus for concern, particularly 'over-consumption of rich food and wines' as well as alcoholic and even sexual 'dissipation'.[95] Ian Miller has argued that there is a 'longstanding tradition' of highlighting the stomach's importance 'to medical, social and cultural life', and certainly it featured frequently in relation to nervous conditions in self-help books.[96] However, any activity which was carried out to excess, 'Over-anxiety, over-work, over-excitement, over-worry', was potentially damaging.[97] What was needed was moderation, and, according to Klickmann, 'order and routine', which would save time and simplify life thus eliminating the chaos and disorder which could provoke nervous suffering.[98]

For some, however, it was not quite so simple as applying the principles of moderation. For several authors suggested that a propensity to nervousness might be hereditary, reflecting concerns about heredity, disease and degeneration that were common at the time. Thus, some people were 'born nervous', while 'nervous breakdown in many cases can be traced to similar disorder in the parents or forefathers of the victim'.[99] Such pronouncements might be interpreted as veiled allusions to congenital venereal disease, as estimates in 1930 suggested as many as 2.6 million patients were suffering from syphilis or gonorrhoea, which although treatable could affect offspring.[100] Ironically, during the nineteenth century syphilis had sometimes been associated with high status and genius among the avant-garde: this was no longer the case.[101] The concern with heredity can also be seen within the context of worries about degeneration, partly prompted by the poor health of volunteers in the Boer and First World Wars but also supported by nascent understandings of genetics and the rise of eugenics in the early decades of the twentieth century.[102] The dangers of such a predisposition were such that as late as the 1950s there were self-help books that recommended men seek heredity counselling if they knew of nervous illness in their family and were thinking of marriage and children.[103]

The causes discussed so far demonstrate the diversity offered and the wide range of human experiences that self-help authors were trying to address. Clearly inherent class and gender assumptions informed authors' explanations. Consistent among the authors was an assumption that many nervous conditions resulted from the individual's choices and lifestyle. On the one hand, this was positive as it conceded agency and an ability to address these factors, both of which were surely intrinsic to self-help books. However, it could also imply that the reader was the architect of his or her own nervousness, and thus alienate the sufferer from the author's positive intent. Equally, it tended to deny the economic, social and political external factors which might cause or contribute to the reader's distress. Authors needed to find a balance as external factors might be far beyond the reader's control and emphasising them might provoke a sense of helplessness. At the same time, they also needed to avoid undermining the reader's sense of personal responsibility for their individual actions.

Ash mentioned the 'poor circumstances, and the innumerable worries associated therewith' that affected 'the less-favoured ranks of society', saying that some of his worst cases were patients of this class. While it might have been a relief for his patients (and readers) to be told that their nervous conditions were not self-inflicted, the limited potential for changing the external circumstances that Ash was ascribing as causes might have been equally distressing.[104] The distinctions and contradictions between external and internal causes illustrate the complexity for author and reader alike of trying to explain a condition which could incorporate so many varying experiences. Although the influence of particular social and cultural beliefs can be seen in some of the causes suggested, ultimately there was no single, clear and simple popular explanation of what caused nervous suffering. Because of this, multiple meanings and understandings could emerge serving different people for differing purposes.

Treatment

While the treatments proposed by self-help authors offered a remarkable level of consistency and continuity in giving agency and control to the reader, they also revealed some inherent contradictions. Undoubtedly, these arose partly because authors were trying to appeal to a wide range of readers by offering a mixture of treatments, but they also reflected the very real difficulty faced in trying to suggest simple solutions to a multiplicity of complex conditions. Treatments tended to fall into three main categories of the physical, behavioural and psychological, but these did not necessarily reflect the same categories of causation or symptoms. Thus, psychological causes and symptoms might be treated with physical remedies and vice versa.

The predominance of digestion as both cause and symptom of nervous conditions led to much focus on diet as a treatment. Klickmann exhorted readers to 'Drink as much hot milk as you can take – you can scarcely take too much', and enthusiastically recommended eating as many as four eggs a day.[105] Most authors recommended moderation and warned against hurrying meals. Contemporary food fashions were revealed in the recommendation of certain foods ('sugar in all forms is a splendid nerve-food, is pleasant to take, and is easily carried about in portable form', suggested Ash).[106] Others counselled against any fastidiousness ('DON'T be over careful in what you eat – unless there are special physical reasons. *Don't be a faddist about food*').[107] Any benefit arising from dietary treatments was most likely a result of the placebo effect, but at the very least such recommendations allowed for reader agency. For those who could afford it, adjustments to diet were easy treatments to implement and eating to restore balance in nervous energy made sense within the popular neurasthenic framework of the early twentieth century.

Another component of restoring deficient nervous energy centred on rest and relaxation and was predicated on the assumption that these were available to the reader. Although the extremes of enforced bed rest which featured in nineteenth-century treatments for neurasthenia had largely disappeared in the twentieth century, having enough rest was considered important. Thus Ash recommended that rest and sleep were vital in stopping the 'worry wheel'. A day off work or 'an extra long night's sleep with breakfast in bed and an easy morning's work to follow' or a long weekend with a change of scene could all 'strengthen the nerves and get rid of the worrying tendencies'.[108] Along with sleep, relaxation was a key treatment for many authors: Edmund Jacobson's whole book, *You Must Relax*, published in 1934, was dedicated to it, and despite his initial reluctance to produce a popular book based on his medical research, it was reprinted several times over the whole century.[109] His approach was very much a physical one and involved learning specific techniques for relaxing muscles and adapting normal everyday postures and movements to a more relaxed style. Like diet, this sort of treatment was straightforward for sufferers to adopt and gave them something active to do about their nervousness, while the underlying rationale that physical relaxation would promote a similar mental state had an appealing logic.

Also logical, for those attributing their nervous conditions to overwork and overindulgence, was the emphasis on exercise, fresh air and getting out of the city. Fresh air and exercise were key elements of contemporary thinking about health, reflected in organisations such as the Women's League of Health and Beauty which had over 170,000 members in Britain by 1939.[110] By the early 1930s, there were half a million hikers and rambling was becoming 'the mass sport of working-class youth'.[111] It was unsurprising therefore that being outdoors and walking featured in many recommended treatments. Walton was specific in prescribing that 'every healthy adult should walk at least two miles daily in the open', while Loosmore considered that 'too much importance cannot be attached to fresh air. This is especially important at the very beginning of nerve trouble.'[112] Other ideas included deep-breathing exercises, cycling and even golf, while outdoor and indoor 'air baths' were a more unusual option.[113] Although outdoor was preferable, the indoor was perhaps easier to achieve without offending the neighbours. This 'simply means removing all your clothes in your own bedroom so as to let the fresh air, which is coming in through the open windows, play upon your body', advised Powell.[114] The more conventional types of bathing involved in water treatments were also a popular suggested treatment, ranging from cold baths, showers and brisk rub-downs to more sophisticated hydrotherapy.[115] Water treatments in the form of visits to spas and taking the waters had a long (and still continuing) history among the wealthy and indeed the kind of hydrotherapy treatments advocated by Powell as proprietor of a 'Nature Cure Health Home' were clearly only available to the well-off.

Several authors emphasised the need for a simple change of scene, and while Klickmann recommended a 'long sea voyage', she was also realistic enough to recognise that not everyone could afford this, offering the simpler alternative to 'get out into the country, if you possibly can, even though you merely take a ride on the top of a bus that is going out among the fields and hedges'.[116] Such advice was consistent with the increasing fashion for and availability of outdoor recreation, day trips and holidays to the country during the interwar period.[117] Loosmore suggested that it was 'impossible to be sad and introspective for long in natural conditions', but then warned against the dangers of going into the country as the quietness might encourage introspection.[118] Such contradictions were rife, as Ash first warned against taking a trip to the seaside as 'the very worst place for people whose nerves are really troublesome', but then argued that for a 'mild case' of nerves a journey to the seaside could be good.[119] The contemporary middle-class understanding that a holiday was largely intended for the benefit of health, rather than the pursuit of enjoyment, was evident in these recommendations, but only Klickmann appeared to address the fact that this might not always be a viable option for her readers.[120] Remedies involving fresh air, holidays, exercise and water were very much focused on the external, physical body despite being aimed at treating the mind. In this way, they again distanced the sufferer from any hint of mental instability and their adoption might easily be explained to others without any unnecessary reference to psychological suffering. Notably none of the recommended water treatments involved medicinal taking of the waters. However, ingested remedies were also featured in self-help books, albeit with some caveats.

Advice with regard to tonics, medicines and drugs fits with the acknowledged narrative of increasing use of pharmacological treatments for mental illness occurring mostly after the Second World War.[121] Before then many sedatives and stimulants were available over the counter, without prescription, which may be why authors in the early century cautioned against them ('far better than soaking the body in nerve tonics and sedatives, or pursuing it with hypodermic injections, is the natural way of simple diet, fresh air, mental rest and proper exercise').[122] Certainly their caution reflected ongoing professional concerns about self-medication. Klickmann specifically singled out patent remedies as not only a hindrance to recovery but also a potential cause of 'undermined' nerves.[123] Sleeping tablets were particularly reviled, Bisch warning his readers never to 'take to sedative drugs' and Ash counselling that 'one hour of natural sleep is at any time worth twelve hours of drugged sleep'.[124] Perhaps the key concern was the risk of readers self-dosing without medical supervision. As few of the self-help authors specifically recommended readers consult a doctor (hardly surprising when their book was supposed to offer a tangible alternative), this was a real concern. Thus, the strong aversion to medicines and drugs in the books reveals the balance self-help authors sought in offering safe and practical treatments without recommending their reader to take advice elsewhere, potentially undermining their authority.

Considering other substances to which readers might resort, most of the authors were distinctly anti-alcohol, particularly in the early century, perhaps influenced by lingering Victorian notions of temperance, and concerns about the stimulant properties of alcohol. 'The safe road both for men and women suffering from nervous ills, is to flee alcohol entirely, since alcohol affects not only the brain, but the nervous system generally', explained Loosmore in 1920.[125] Tobacco was also frowned upon, considered by some as a poison and 'often a serious factor in some forms of nervous ailments'. However, others argued, 'there is considerable agreement that tobacco, even in nerve strain, may not be harmful, where it is indulged in, in strict moderation'.[126] Both comments came long before the real harmfulness of smoking was known, but illustrate the contradictory nature of much advice around everyday substances. Similarly, tea and coffee were problematised by some.[127] The removal of alcohol, tea, coffee and smoking as sources of pleasure might imply a somewhat miserable regime. However, authors were also at pains to ensure that sufferers engaged in activities that were enjoyable.

Many considered play and enjoyment as significant in treating nervous disorders, thus the anonymous author of *From Terror to Triumph* warned, 'To sit in a corner and mope is extremely harmful' and recommended filling the mind 'with pleasant thoughts and concentrate on something outside yourself'.[128] Powell in 1926 recommended, 'Lectures, provided they are not about Egyptian Mummies or some other equally doleful subject, form another useful means of uplift', and 'Sermons, too, help if your preacher be an optimist!'[129] For many reading was an important source of cheer with Browning and Burns's poetry and the works of Robert Louis Stevenson and *Punch* magazine commended for inspiring a 'mood of hope and courage and good cheer'.[130] Certain reading matter was to be avoided ('if you read a newspaper when you are ill (not always advisable by any means) omit all the records of crime, vice and other unpleasantness', warned Klickmann). However, returning 'to your old favourites when the brain is weary or the system below par' was a good idea.[131]

The general message was simple. According to Ash, recreation was a 'very important part of the self-help programme', while Powell was more emphatic, insisting that 'Hobbies help to preserve our youth and sanity.'[132] Proposed hobbies ranged from playing a musical instrument, sketching or painting to jigsaw puzzles.[133] Unlike work, concentrating on a hobby was safe. 'Don't be afraid of working your mind: you can't overwork it, provided of course, that the work is congenial and absorbs your interest', suggested one author. However, others warned against chess and games 'in which the excitements of gambling are a conspicuous feature', as these were too taxing.[134] The focus on hobbies reflected a growing awareness of occupational therapy, rather than rest cures, and the benefits of distracting the sufferer from their condition.[135] However, the extent to which issues of class or gender were taken into consideration by these authors seems negligible, as a struggling working-class mother might only have dreamed of enough time and resources for a hobby.

Physical treatments focused mainly on rest, relaxation, fresh air, exercise and managing diet and legal stimulants, with the addition of more faddish or exclusive treatments such as hydrotherapy. None of these represented new ideas about treating ill-health, but their application to the treatment of nervous conditions saw them offered in a new context. To some extent, all were likely to be available, in some form, to the self-help reader and so were advised by many authors hopeful of providing practical solutions, but also with an eye to attracting readers. Expensive and/or exclusive treatments were unlikely to have wide appeal and were self-defeating in self-help books, most of which were written with the intention that the reader could carry out their own treatment. Unsurprisingly the same general approach was also applied by authors to the potentially more complex question of psychological treatments.

Psychological approaches to treatment were often couched in physical terms, so authors recommended the reader bring their psyche back under control through training. Framing treatment in this way placed it firmly within a physical exercise paradigm or the more acceptable psychological framework of Pelmanism, a particular enthusiasm of the early decades of the twentieth century.[136] Hence Powell in the 1920s put his emphasis on 'nerve training', in his book *How to Train Your Nerves: A Manual of Nerve Training*.[137] Other authors reported that exercising the 'powers of attention or concentration is clear proof of mind-control', and suggested various practices to achieve this, such as practising observation, because, 'By observing others, you forget yourself.'[138]

Such exercises were intended to give the sufferer a sense of agency and control, particularly relevant to those who feared that their nerves were somehow out of control, with the implication that carried of impending madness. Carrying out simple observation exercises would at the very least give them some tangible sense of progress or improvement. In a similar vein, authors encouraged their readers to adopt 'right thinking' through exercising self-discipline and will power. Ash explained what this meant: 'bright and optimistic thoughts are helpful whilst pessimistic and dismal thoughts are bad for our nerves', adding that this was 'so obvious that one scarcely need refer to it except to illustrate the whole idea of right-thinking'.[139] Contemporaries such as Loosmore advocated self-discipline: 'Much may be said for the practice of forcing oneself to do things, occasionally, which are disagreeable and opposed to one's natural inclinations', while the anonymous author of *From Terror to Triumph* advised, '*Practise self-control. Deny yourself an indulgence occasionally – it strengthens.*'[140] This emphasis on self-control, self-denial and discipline fitted within the paradigm of health, fitness and training, but also within social norms that emphasised emotional control and stoicism.

Such norms were also reflected in advice to readers about their general attitude to life and particularly the benefits of religious faith. Cheerfulness was considered important, so developing a sense of humour and with it, importantly, a sense of perspective was advocated by many: 'Cheerfulness must be cultivated and maintained by reading cheerful books, and thus, as in other ways, keeping in touch with cheerful people.'[141] Klickmann counselled readers to 'resolve to live only a day at a time – actually *one day at a time*', and recommended half an hour's complete silence per day, explaining, 'surely every woman is entitled to at least one half-hour to herself out of the twenty-four, for quiet conversation with her own soul'.[142] Notably, her recommended practices were still being highlighted in so-called mindfulness approaches at the end of the century.[143] The soul was a key feature for many authors, several of them suggesting sufferers turn to God.[144] Loosmore advised that religion was needed to supplement psychology, as 'faith in the ultimate and the unseen' eased the strain of living and generated hope.[145] Reflecting the same contemporary enthusiasm for drawing on many forms of the unknown, Ash argued it would be a mistake to be content with orthodox psychology and ignore the 'greater possibilities that lie before us in the unexplored field of the occult'.[146] Unfortunately, he did not expand further on quite how the occult might practically help, but his views reflected the fact that for many at the time, the concept of the unconscious was consistent with occult notions of the untapped potential of the mind.[147] Indeed, Spiritualism, which enjoyed a period of considerable popularity during the interwar period, assimilated both psychological and psychoanalytical concepts into its own eclectic practice, so his comment was not unusual.[148]

Such concepts also informed some recommended treatments. Ash and Schofield both discussed the use of auto-suggestion to influence the subconscious, identifying poor self-control, 'painful or distressing nerve-body reactions', lack of poise and self-confidence, and low spirits as suitable for correction in this way.[149] Bisch recommended acting on fears and building up resistance to nerve-inducing events, through repeated exposure. 'Shock yourself often in a vicarious manner and you won't be so shocked when the unexpected of a frightening or even harrowing nature occurs in real life', he proposed, adding that for sources of the unexpected, 'mystery and detective stories are excellent'.[150] Bisch's suggestion was effectively a forerunner of the kind of behaviourist desensitising exposure therapy developed later in the century by Joseph Wolpe (1915–1997), but it could hardly have sat well with his contemporaries who advocated no exciting reading matter for sufferers.[151] In one of the rare recommendations to elicit professional help, Powell, in the mid-1920s, advised, 'look into your mental or psychic life. Or, better still let a trained psychologist or psycho-analyst look into it along with you.'[152] Although there was some mention of doctors and advice to consult them, this was, unsurprisingly, relatively rare as self-help books existed to enable readers to avoid such a consultation. The most notable absence therefore in the books was any great exhortation for the sufferer to share their problems or for the therapeutic value of talking. Instead, the overriding sense was of suffering with discretion. This contrasts hugely with the late twentieth-century obsession with sharing one's problems, whether in therapy or, increasingly towards the end of the century, in public on national television.[153]

Conclusion

The early twentieth century saw the development of popular interest in psychology reflected in the growing success of self-help books. The books examined in this chapter were concerned with the diagnosis and treatment of nervous conditions and intended to enable sufferers from mental distress to self-diagnose and treat their conditions. Aimed at a lay audience, for the most part, they were written in non-technical language and often employed vernacular terminology reflecting authorial conversations with patients. This was consistent with the popular enthusiasm for practical psychology which emphasised self-improvement and focused the reader on issues of self-responsibility, choice and control. Mental illness and psychological suffering continued to be stigmatised during this period, despite greater popular awareness of psychological problems resulting from the First World War and increased interest in the realms of the psychological seen in such features as advice columns in newspapers. Suffering from nerves was still something to be discreet about, and thus many of the books privileged physical symptoms to reassure readers worried about insanity or afraid of the taint of mental ill-health. Most self-help books were written by and for a middle-class, educated audience and class and gender assumptions inherent in discussions of causes and treatments reflected this fact. Fundamental to such books was a belief in human agency that saw the reader as able and empowered to improve their own condition. The potential downside to such a philosophy was the effective overlooking of any other environmental or social issues which might be causes of problems or require addressing to enable improvement. By its nature, the self-help book could only work on the subject of the problem rather than their wider context. Yet it was often the environment and circumstances in which people found themselves that appeared to be the problem. Indeed, a common theme was the threat posed by modern life, particularly lifestyle choices, technology, speed and social change. This apparent dichotomy of focusing on the inherent flaw of the individual rather than addressing external circumstances would underpin the approach to nervous conditions and stress for much of the coming century.

Notes

1 Edwin Lancelot Hopewell Ash, *On Keeping Our Nerves in Order* (London: Mills & Boon, 1928), pp. 8–9. Ash was a prolific writer on nervous diseases and worked at various times at the Kensington and Fulham General Hospital, the West End Nerve Hospital and at St Mary's Hospital, Paddington.

2 Thomson, *Psychological Subjects*, p. 179.
3 For a more detailed history of the development of popular psychology see Thomson's *Psychological Subjects*. Pelmanism was, among other things, a memory training programme. Although Thomson suggests the height of Pelmanism's popularity was the early decades of the twentieth century, an advert for the Pelman Institute and its courses appeared in 1950 in a self-help book by John Kennedy, *Worry: Its Cause and Cure* (London: The Psychologist, 1950), suggesting its popularity persisted somewhat longer.
4 Richard Overy, *The Morbid Age: Britain and the Crisis of Civilization 1919–1939* (London: Penguin, 2010), p. 6.
5 Barham, *Forgotten Lunatics*, p. 4.
6 *Ibid.*, p. 5; Thomson, *Psychological Subjects*, p. 185; Loughran, 'Shell-Shock', p. 91.
7 Fiona Reid, *Broken Men: Shell Shock, Treatment and Recovery in Britain 1914–1930* (London; New York: Continuum, 2010), p. 10. Dorothy L. Sayers, *The Unpleasantness at the Bellona Club* (London: Ernest Benn, 1928).
8 Overy, *Morbid Age*, p. 13.
9 Sally Alexander, 'Men's Fears and Women's Work: Responses to Unemployment in London between the Wars', *Gender & History* 12, 2 (2000): pp. 407–10, http://dx.doi.org/10.1111/1468-0424.00189.
10 Overy, *Morbid Age*, p. 20.
11 Thomson, *Psychological Subjects*, pp. 51–2, 209; Richards, 'Britain on the Couch', p. 204.
12 Thomson, *Psychological Subjects*, pp. 50–2.
13 The sample resulted from a search of the British Library catalogue using a wide range of synonyms for stress. I then selected books that were explicitly aimed at a popular audience, deducing this from authors' statements on dust jackets or in prefaces and on the language used and contents listed.
14 Thomson, 'Neurasthenia', p. 81.
15 David G. Schuster, *Neurasthenic Nation: America's Search for Health, Happiness and Comfort, 1869–1920* (London: Rutgers University Press, 2011), pp. 159–60.
16 C. W. Saleeby, *Worry: The Disease of the Age* (London; Paris; New York; Melbourne: Cassell & Co. Ltd, 1907); George Lincoln Walton, *Why Worry?* (Philadelphia; London: J. B. Lippincott Co., 1908); Alfred Taylor Schofield, *Nervousness: A Brief and Popular Review of the Moral Treatment of Disordered Nerves* (London: William Rider & Sons Ltd, 1910); Edwin Lancelot Hopewell Ash, *Nerves and the Nervous* (London: Mills & Boon,

1911); Edwin Lancelot Hopewell Ash, *The Problem of Nervous Breakdown* (London: Mills & Boon, 1919).

17 Jackson, *Age of Stress*, pp. 34–7.

18 Overy, *Morbid Age*, p. 175.

19 For example, Louis Edward Bisch, *Be Glad You're Neurotic* (New York: McGraw-Hill, 1936), p. 156. For a detailed chronological history of the science and medicine of stress, see Jackson, *Age of Stress*.

20 Rapp, 'Reception of Freud', p. 219.

21 Overy, *Morbid Age*, p. 148.

22 Christine B. Whelan, 'Self-Help Books and the Quest for Self-Control in the United States 1950–2000' (PhD thesis, University of Oxford, 2004), p. 21; Sue Currell, 'Depression and Recovery: Self-Help and America in the 1930s', in David Bell and Joanne Hollows (eds) *Historicizing Lifestyle: Mediating Taste, Consumption and Identity from the 1900s to 1970s* (Aldershot: Ashgate Publishing Ltd, 2006), p. 133; Steven Starker, 'Promises and Prescriptions: Self-Help Books in Mental Health and Medicine', *American Journal of Health Promotion* 1, 2 (1 September 1986): p. 20, https://doi.org/10.4278/0890-1171-1.2.19.

23 Currell, 'Depression and Recovery', p. 134.

24 Walter Boughton Pitkin, *Life Begins at Forty* (New York: McGraw-Hill, 1932); Walter Boughton Pitkin, *More Power to You! A Working Technique for Making the Most of Human Energy* (Garden City: Garden City Publishing Co., 1933).

25 Whelan, 'Self-Help Books', pp. 33–4; Dale Carnegie, *How to Win Friends and Influence People* (New York: Simon & Schuster, 1937).

26 John Feather, *A History of British Publishing* (London: Croom Helm, 1988), p. 203.

27 Bisch, *Neurotic*; David Harold Fink, *Release from Nervous Tension* (London: George Allen and Unwin Ltd, 1946).

28 Iain Stevenson, *Book Makers: British Publishing in the Twentieth Century* (London: The British Library, 2010), p. 73.

29 Examples include: Milton R. Powell, *How to Train Your Nerves: A Manual of Nerve Training* (London: Lutterworth Press, 1926), 4 pp.; William Drummond Kendall, *The Conquest of Nerves* (London: St Clements Press, 1932), 32 pp.; Ernest White, *Overcoming Fears and Worries* (Watford: C&A Simpson Ltd, 1945), 20 pp.

30 Frank Arthur Mumby and Ian Norrie, *Mumby's Publishing and Bookselling in the 20th Century* (London: Bell & Hyman, 1982), p. 221.

31 Alfred Taylor Schofield, *Nerves in Disorder: A Plea for Rational Treatment* (New York; London: Funk & Wagnells, 1903); Edmund Jacobson, *You*

Must Relax: A Practical Method of Reducing the Strains of Modern Living (New York; London: McGraw-Hill Book Co., 1934).

32 Brief mention of shell shock or war can be found in: William Charles Loosmore, *Nerves and the Man: A Popular Psychological and Constructive Study of Nervous Breakdown* (London: John Murray, 1922), pp. 44–5; Ash, *Nerves in Order*, p. 8. Two chapters on the effects of war strain and shell shock are in Ash, *Nervous Breakdown*.

33 Ash, *Nerves in Order*, p. 8; Loosmore, *Nerves*, pp. 44–5.

34 Ash, *Nerves and the Nervous*, preface.

35 Dougall MacDougall King, *Nerves and Personal Power: Some Principles of Psychology as Applied to Conduct and Health* (London: George Allen & Unwin, 1923), preface; Schofield, *Nerves in Disorder*, preface.

36 Josephine A. Jackson and Helen M. Salisbury, *Outwitting Our Nerves: A Primer of Psychotherapy*, 3rd ed. (London: Kegan Paul, Trench, Trubner, 1927), foreword.

37 Kendall, *Conquest of Nerves*, preface.

38 Bisch, *Neurotic*, p. 31.

39 Flora Klickmann, *Mending Your Nerves* (London: RTS, 1925); Powell, *Train Your Nerves*.

40 Kendall, *Conquest of Nerves*; Jackson and Salisbury, *Outwitting Our Nerves*.

41 Rapp, 'The Reception of Freud', p. 198.

42 George Lincoln Watson, *Those Nerves* (New York: Simple Life Series, 1910); Orison Swett Marden, *Making Friends with Our Nerves* (New York: T. Y. Crowell Co., 1925).

43 Loosmore, *Nerves*.

44 Whelan, 'Self-Help Books', p. 7.

45 Overy, *Morbid Age*, p. 168.

46 Bisch, *Neurotic*, p. 73.

47 Anne Digby, *The Evolution of British General Practice, 1850–1948* (Oxford: Oxford University Press, 1999), p. 307. 'Replies to Spring Directive You and the NHS' (1997), MOA, University of Sussex, N1592 and A706.

48 Loosmore, *Nerves*, 18; Milton R. Powell, *The Safe Way to Sound Nerves by Rational Nature Cure Drugless Methods* (London: Lutterworth Press, 1926), p. 5.

49 Rhodri Hayward, 'Busman's Stomach 1937: Digestive Disorders and the Making of Modern Politics', *History of Emotions – Insights into Research*, 2015, https://doi.org/DOI:10.14280/08241.36; Edgar Jones, '"The Gut War": Functional Somatic Disorders in the UK during the

Second World War', *History of the Human Sciences* 25, 5 (1 December 2012): p. 31, https://doi.org/10.1177/0952695112466515.

50 Bisch, *Neurotic*, p. 142; Klickmann, *Mending Your Nerves*, p. 112.
51 Powell, *Train Your Nerves*, p. 7; 'A Specialist', *From Terror to Triumph: How to Fight and Conquer Neurasthenia, Insomnia and Other Nervous Disorders* (Epsom: E. G. Pullinger, 1932), pp. 7–8.
52 'A Specialist', *Terror*, p. 8; Loosmore, *Nerves*, p. 17; Klickmann, *Mending Your Nerves*, p. 112.
53 Ash, *Nerves and the Nervous*, pp. 2, 13–14; Loosmore, *Nerves*, p. 21.
54 Loosmore, *Nerves*, pp. 13–14; Powell, *Sound Nerves*, p. 38.
55 Loosmore, *Nerves*, p. 21; 'A Specialist', *Terror*, p. 7.
56 Bisch, *Neurotic*, p. 6.
57 Loosmore, *Nerves*, pp. 15, 19.
58 Schofield, *Nervousness*, p. 28.
59 'A Specialist', *Terror*, p. 17. Italics in the original.
60 Overy, *Morbid Age*, pp. 3–4.
61 Alexander, 'Men's Fears', pp. 406, 408.
62 Overy, *Morbid Age*, pp. 314–15.
63 Loosmore, *Nerves*, p. 21.
64 Schofield, *Nervousness*, p. 9.
65 Overy, *Morbid Age*, p. 98.
66 For the history of eugenics in Britain see Mathew Thomson, *The Problem of Mental Deficiency: Eugenics, Democracy and Social Policy in Britain c. 1870–1959* (Oxford: Oxford University Press, 1998).
67 Jon Turney, *Frankenstein's Footsteps: Science, Genetics and Popular Culture* (New Haven: Yale University Press, 1998), pp. 59–62; Jim Endersby, *A Guinea Pig's History of Biology* (London: Arrow Books, 2008), p. 176.
68 Ash, *Nerves and the Nervous*, pp. 5–6.
69 Ash, *Nerves in Order*, p. 37.
70 Ash, *Nerves and the Nervous*, p. 52.
71 Hayward, 'Busman's Stomach'.
72 Ash, *Nerves and the Nervous*, p. 2; Schofield, *Nervousness*, p. 10.
73 Walter Beran Wolfe, *Nervous Breakdown: Its Cause and Cure* (New York: Farrar & Rinehart, 1933), p. 12.
74 Jackson, *Age of Stress*, pp. 14–15; Cooper and Dewe, *Stress*, pp. 2–3; Wainwright and Calnan, *Work Stress*, p. 37.
75 Currell, 'Depression and Recovery', p. 135.
76 Loosmore, *Nerves*, p. 32.
77 Ash, *Nerves in Order*, p. 25.
78 Bisch, *Neurotic*, p. 11.
79 Loosmore, *Nerves*, p. 3.

80 Bisch, *Neurotic*, p. 3.
81 Ash, *Nerves and the Nervous*, pp. 66–7.
82 Bisch, *Neurotic*, p. 42; Walton, *Why Worry?* pp. 245–6.
83 Ash, *Nerves and the Nervous*, p. 51.
84 Klickmann, *Mending Your Nerves*, p. 19.
85 Oppenheim, *Shattered Nerves*, pp. 181–2.
86 Walton, *Why Worry?* pp. 260–1.
87 Ash, *Nerves and the Nervous*, p. 40; Stephen Taylor, 'The Suburban Neurosis', *The Lancet* 231, 5978 (1938): p. 759, https://doi.org/10.1016/S0140-6736(00)93869-8; Frederick Cooper, 'Medical Feminism, Working Mothers, and the Limits of Home: Finding a Balance between Self-Care and Other-Care in Cross-Cultural Debates about Health and Lifestyle, 1952–1956', *Palgrave Communications* 2 (2016): pp. 3–5, https://doi.org/10.1057/palcomms.2016.42; Betty Friedan, *The Feminine Mystique* (New York: W. W. Norton, 1963).
88 Schofield, *Nervousness*, p. 38.
89 Klickmann, *Mending Your Nerves*, p. 37.
90 *Ibid.*, p. 95.
91 *Ibid.*, p. 21.
92 Penny Summerfield, *Women Workers in the Second World War: Production and Patriarchy in Conflict* (London: Routledge, 1989), p. 123; Cooper, 'Medical Feminism', p. 3; 'Can Women Take the Pressure?', *The Times* (17 February 1982), p. 15.
93 Loosmore, *Nerves*, p. 45.
94 Ash, *Nerves and the Nervous*, pp. 40–1; Loosmore, *Nerves*, p. 46; Powell, *Sound Nerves*, p. 4.
95 Ash, *Nerves and the Nervous*, pp. 40–1; Powell, *Sound Nerves*, p. 4.
96 Ian Miller, *A Modern History of the Stomach: Gastric Illness, Medicine and British Society, 1800–1950.* (Abingdon, Oxon: Routledge, 2016), pp. 1–2.
97 Klickmann, *Mending Your Nerves*, p. 17.
98 *Ibid.*, p. 116.
99 Schofield, *Nervousness*, p. 36; Loosmore, *Nerves*, p. 24.
100 Overy, *Morbid Age*, p. 153.
101 Roy Porter, *The Greatest Benefit to Mankind: A Medical History of Humanity from Antiquity to the Present* (London: Fontana Press, 1999), p. 451.
102 Endersby, *Guinea Pig's History*, p. 176; Turney, *Frankenstein's Footsteps*, p. 59.
103 Walter C. Alvarez, *Live At Peace with Your Nerves* (Englewood Cliffs: Prentice-Hall, 1958), p. 109.
104 Ash, *Nerves and the Nervous*, p. 51.

105 Klickmann, *Mending Your Nerves*, p. 24.
106 Ash, *Nerves and the Nervous*, p. 207.
107 'A Specialist', *Terror*, p. 19. Italics in the original.
108 Ash, *Nerves in Order*, p. 53.
109 Jacobson, *You Must Relax*, p. 51; Loosmore, *Nerves*, pp. 55–7.
110 Jill Julius Matthews, 'They Had Such a Lot of Fun: The Women's League of Health and Beauty between the Wars', *History Workshop Journal* 30, 1 (21 September 1990): p. 23, https://doi.org/10.1093/hwj/30.1.22.
111 Ben Harker, '"The Manchester Rambler": Ewan MacColl and the 1932 Mass Trespass', *History Workshop Journal* 59, 1 (2005): p. 220, https://doi.org/10.1093/hwj/dbi016.
112 Walton, *Why Worry?* p. 256; Loosmore, *Nerves*, pp. 80–1.
113 Loosmore, *Nerves*, pp. 78–80; Powell, *Train Your Nerves*, p. 24.
114 Powell, *Train Your Nerves*, p. 24.
115 Walton, *Why Worry?* p. 255; Bisch, *Neurotic*, pp. 109–10; Powell, *Train Your Nerves*, p. 28.
116 Klickmann, *Mending Your Nerves*, pp. 33–4, 50.
117 R. J. Moore-Colyer, 'From Great Wen to Toad Hall: Aspects of the Urban–Rural Divide in Inter-War Britain', *Rural History* 10, 1 (1999): p. 113, https://doi.org/10.1017/S0956793300001710.
118 Loosmore, *Nerves*, pp. 49, 58.
119 Ash, *Nerves and the Nervous*, p. 193.
120 Susan Barton, *Working-Class Organisations and Popular Tourism, 1840–1970* (Manchester: Manchester University Press, 2005), pp. 73–4; Klickmann, *Mending Your Nerves*, p. 50.
121 Jordan Goodman, 'Pharmaceutical Industry', in Cooter and Pickstone (eds) *Companion to Medicine*, p. 148.
122 Healy, *Prozac*, p. 4; Ash, *Nerves in Order*, p. 43.
123 Klickmann, *Mending Your Nerves*, p. 105.
124 Bisch, *Neurotic*, pp. 109–10; Ash, *Nerves and the Nervous*, p. 166.
125 Loosmore, *Nerves*, p. 86.
126 Ash, *Nerves and the Nervous*, pp. 213–14; Loosmore, *Nerves*, p. 84.
127 Powell, *Sound Nerves*, p. 37.
128 'A Specialist', *Terror*, p. 21.
129 Powell, *Sound Nerves*, p. 41.
130 *Ibid.*; Loosmore, *Nerves*, pp. 126–8.
131 Klickmann, *Mending Your Nerves*, pp. 62, 65.
132 Ash, *Nerves and the Nervous*, p. 191; Powell, *Sound Nerves*, p. 41.
133 Loosmore, *Nerves*, p. 57; Klickmann, *Mending Your Nerves*, p. 131.
134 'A Specialist', *Terror*, p. 21; Ash, *Nerves and the Nervous*, p. 191.
135 Ben Harris and Courtney Stevens, 'From Rest Cure to Work Cure', *Monitor on Psychology* 41, 5 (2010): pp. 26–7.

136 Thomson, *Psychological Subjects*, pp. 23–4.

137 Powell, *Train Your Nerves*, pp. 5–6.

138 Ash, *Nerves and the Nervous*, pp. 158–9; 'A Specialist', *Terror*, p. 16.

139 Ash, *Nerves in Order*, p. 84.

140 Loosmore, *Nerves*, p. 159; 'A Specialist', *Terror*, p. 16. Italics in the original.

141 Wolfe, *Nervous Breakdown: Its Cause and Cure*, p. 221; Loosmore, *Nerves*, p. 125.

142 Klickmann, *Mending Your Nerves*, pp. 77, 126. Italics in the original.

143 Jon Kabat-Zinn, *Full Catastrophe Living: Using the Wisdom of Your Body and Mind to Face Stress, Pain and Illness* (New York: Delacorte Press, 1990), p. 19.

144 Loosmore, *Nerves*, p. 57; Klickmann, *Mending Your Nerves*, pp. 135–6; Schofield, *Nerves in Disorder*, p. 171.

145 Loosmore, *Nerves*, p. 117.

146 Ash, *Nerves in Order*, p. 73.

147 Alex Owen, 'Occultism and the "Modern" Self in Fin-de-Siècle Britain', in Martin Daunton and Bernhard Rieger (eds) *Meanings of Modernity: Britain from the Late Victorian Era to World War II* (Oxford: Berg, 2001), p. 77.

148 Jenny Hazelgrove, *Spiritualism and British Society between the Wars* (Manchester: Manchester University Press, 2000), p. 37.

149 Ash, *Nerves in Order*, p. 82; Schofield, *Nerves in Disorder*, p. 123.

150 Bisch, *Neurotic*, p. 177.

151 For a brief explanation of Wolpe's approach see Allan V. Horwitz, *Anxiety: A Short History* (Baltimore, MD: The Johns Hopkins University Press, 2013), pp. 110–11.

152 Powell, *Sound Nerves*, p. 6.

153 Franny Nudelman, 'Beyond the Talking Cure', in Joel Pfister and Nancy Schnog (eds) *Inventing the Psychological: Toward a Cultural History of Emotional Life in America* (New Haven; London: Yale University Press, 1997), p. 310.

2

Neurotic tendencies: workplace and suburban neurosis in the interwar period

In 1930 the Medical Research Council (MRC) published a 'pioneer survey' by its Industrial Health Research Board (IHRB) investigating the prevalence of 'neurotic tendencies' in the British workforce with particular focus on 'imperfect mental adaptation to conditions of work' and how it reduced 'working efficiency'.[1] Such research was ambitious, aimed at clarifying specific organisational problems, including: 'absenteeism through sickness labelled "nervous breakdown" or one of its synonyms'; selection for promotion of individuals able to direct 'without undue strain to themselves'; and erratic workers doing 'very good and very bad work for no apparent reason'.[2] As the mention of synonyms suggests, the researchers were aware that they were dealing with a set of conditions with many different labels (nervous breakdown, strain, neurotic tendencies) that were subjectively applied. Whether the worker believed himself or herself 'nervy' or under too much 'strain', the absenteeism and underperformance that such conditions created reduced an organisation's efficiency and productivity. The IHRB researchers were also interested in why 'indifferent environmental conditions' could cause 'disproportionate suffering' to some, but not to others.[3] However, while environment was understood as the context for this question, the focus was on the individual's response, rather than on the potential harmfulness of the environment itself.

Raising similar questions about environment and failure to adapt in another context at much the same time was Stephen Taylor, a doctor at the Royal Free Hospital in Hampstead, north London. He was concerned about the effect on women of moving from inner-city housing to new suburban estates such as the Watling estate in Hendon on the outskirts of London. Taylor identified a new, psychological complaint specific to these women that he called 'suburban neurosis', and which arguably echoed the focus of the IHRB study, as it too appeared to result from an imperfect mental adaptation: in this case to the conditions of suburban life.[4] Broader concerns about the health of the poor living in London prompted an experiment in Peckham that came to similar conclusions, albeit its subjects were decidedly urban.[5] In all of these studies, despite the apparent relevance of environmental factors to nervous suffering, and in Taylor's case, the reference to specific geography in the actual name of the complaint, conclusions tended to emphasise the inherent weakness of the individual. This was consistent with contemporary popular thinking reflected in the self-help books of the last chapter. It was individual failure to adjust to conditions rather than the nature of those conditions themselves that was the problem in cases of nerves, whether at work or at home.

By exploring these three studies and drawing on retrospective accounts of everyday life in the first half of the twentieth century, this chapter uncovers how stress, under the labels of neurosis and nerves, was constructed by contemporary researchers in both work and domestic settings. In doing so, I also examine people's own explanations for their experiences and the cultural norms that informed them. Early research in organisations, shaped by the growth of scientific management, sought to identify workers susceptible to nervous conditions and to evaluate their impact on productivity, with a view to avoiding their employment or managing them more effectively. Such attempts were largely confounded by the range and inconsistency of worker experiences, arising partly from the very diversity of those experiences, but also because of the complexity of the relationship between worker and work. Personal accounts of work in this period reveal attitudes and beliefs about work based not only on its necessity for survival but also its critical role in identity, status and social life. The complexities of work's meaning informed how people understood experiences of work-related stress, and for many meant that it simply could not be acknowledged, only endured, or hidden behind a physical proxy, and this fitted with an expectation of stoicism that was commonplace at the time.

Equally difficult to acknowledge was the fact that the achievement of a new, sanitary, spacious, suburban home might lead to nervous conditions rather than contentment. Much research into neurosis at work focused on men, but Taylor's suburban neurosis diagnosis referred exclusively to women and effectively pathologised the experiences of many who moved out of the inner-city slums. While housewives reported relief to be living in a new, safe, clean home, away from the physical discomforts of the slums, the move to the modern, new housing estates created its own problems. The experience of home was paradoxical: it was a place that often functioned as a retreat from the pressure and strain of work and the outside world (particularly for men) but was also the location of work and cause of considerable distress, for many women. Such findings by the researchers at the Peckham Health Centre potentially challenged Taylor's designation of 'suburban' to his study of neuroses, as their work revealed similar problems among urban households. Arguably what emerged in both environments was the gendered nature of domestic stress, often underpinned by lack of interaction with the outside world and a privileging of privacy that led to loneliness and isolation. What all three research projects had in common was the idea that some people in certain environments suffered from what they expressed as 'their nerves' and which researchers termed neurosis. In each case, the researchers were trying to establish a way of identifying who would be susceptible and to understand just why they succumbed.

Industrial efficiency

The broader context for the IHRB research into neurotic tendencies in the workplace in the interwar period was the economic impact of the Depression, concerns about mental hygiene and the foundation of industrial psychology following the publication in the USA of Frederick Taylor's seminal monograph *The Principles of Scientific Management* in 1911.[6] Focusing on methods to increase efficiency, it prompted researchers to study how work was managed as well as the impact of different environmental factors in the workplace, with publications such as Elton Mayo's *The Human Problems of Industrial Civilisation* of 1933 producing influential findings on the psychological functioning of workers in the USA.[7] The IHRB itself had begun life as the Industrial Fatigue Research Board created at the end of the First World War to continue the work of the Health of Munitions Workers Committee which had been set up to look at issues of fatigue, health and efficiency in munitions factories.[8] By 1930, its name had changed to reflect its wider remit.

During the interwar years medical discussions about strain in the industrial workplace were largely overshadowed by debates about whether national insurance and compensation laws provided an incentive for malingerers, reflecting an attitude of suspicion rather than concern for worker well-being, focused on malingering and moral weakness.[9] Nevertheless, some employers were developing welfare policies during the period that included some element of health care for workers, although occupational health practices tended to be better developed in nationalised industries than in private concerns.[10] An exception to this, discussed by Ronnie Johnston and Arthur McIvor, was Bilslands Bakers, one of Glasgow's factory bakeries in the interwar period. Bilslands had a 'comprehensive welfarist strategy' including provision of multiple leisure facilities such as summer camps for young workers, gym classes and sports teams as well as having its own doctor, dentist and optician. Such care was not purely altruistic, but also served to ensure a healthy and hygienic workforce, thus reducing sickness absence. It was also consistent with a managerial anti-union policy, highlighting one of the reasons that unions were often deeply suspicious of early welfare practices.[11] Bilslands was, however, more the exception than the rule. Among small to medium-sized companies, worker welfare and health provision were more often limited or non-existent.[12] Much of the research on worker health carried out during this period was focused on the physical rather than the psychological, although studies in the late 1930s did explore links between intelligence, boredom and strain.[13]

It was notable that the project announced by the MRC in 1930, while acknowledging that most previous research by the IHRB had focused on physical conditions of work, such as hours worked, emphasised that this study was taking a more psychological stance in looking at 'mental adaptation to conditions of work' and that its methods were 'somewhat experimental'.[14] These involved researching over a thousand male and female workers, including 'clerical workers in Government departments and commercial firms, factory workers, people in administrative posts, and students' whose ages ranged from fourteen to sixty. The data were based on answers to hypothetical situations posed in relatively unstructured personal interviews and while the findings claimed there was a latent body of nervous workers, they also acknowl-edged difficulties in both recognising who they were and how to quantify the effects of their suffering on their work.[15] The researchers admitted that 'nervous symptoms are of infinite variety and often peculiar to the individual', reflecting the conclusions of the self-help authors in the last chapter. They therefore acknowledged that the focus of their study might encompass a wide range of experiences and labels.

However, despite such 'infinite variety', the authors claimed to have identified two 'recognised clinical types'. The first worker suffered from 'fears connected with authorities, causeless apprehension, irrational worries connected with the work or with the imagined judgements of other people', while the second had an unreasonable drive to dwell on certain thoughts, which if resisted created 'great stress'.[16] The researchers provided specific examples: '1) Woman aged 29; eldest of four. Engaged on routine clerical work and finds it monotonous; can think of other things when at work without affecting it. Had a month off lately for "nerves"; had made a mistake and it worried her.' The same woman would 'feel nervous momentarily' if sent for by a superior and was 'nervous if spoken to by strangers', and would feel faint in trains or crowds, although she attributed this to a weak heart resulting from influenza. Further details of her case also included this mixture of psychological and physical symptoms, such as a feeling 'of something awful going to happen', eye strain and headaches, demonstrating again that people were often more comfortable acknowledging a physical symptom which effectively acted as a proxy for their psychological distress. A further case made direct links between wartime experience and nervous symptoms and suggests a degree of familiarity with similar war-related cases:

> 2. Man of 33. Second of two. In a responsible administrative position. Likes his work very much; wouldn't do work that did not demand his whole attention. Says he is highly strung. Wakes up and thinks about his work. Was on active service and tended to stammer afterwards. His noticeably slow speech, now a fixed habit, was an effort to overcome it ... on being pressed he shows an obvious reluctance to talk of his war experiences (typical of 'post-war neurasthenic').[17]

Both instances are interesting for the contrast between the ordinary person's language and that of the researchers, the woman in the first

case having suffered from 'nerves' and the man in the second calling
himself 'highly strung'. Indeed, the researchers commented on this,
reporting that the workers 'do not call themselves "nervous", though
they may admit to being "nervy"'. Evidently, workers made a distinction
between the more colloquial nomenclature and that of the experts:
being 'highly strung' was preferable to the more medical 'neurasthenic'
or 'neurotic'.[18] Popular terminology was less precise and allowed for
a range of interpretation, although arguably, the medical term 'neurasthenic' was in many respects equally vague.[19]

Despite encountering a range of nervous people and establishing
that it was 'possible to distinguish the nervous person and to diagnose
his type', the researchers were forced to acknowledge that with regard
to any detrimental effect on output 'evidence is difficult to obtain'.[20]
This was because although they established the existence of considerable
numbers of people with nervous conditions, it was hard to distinguish
those who might be destined for long periods of absence from work,
from those able to manage their work despite their suffering.[21] Thus,
it was hard to quantify the connection between nervousness and
productivity as one did not always have a negative effect on the other.
This was not because such workers were not suffering, but rather that
they continued to work despite their nerves.

Although personal accounts from workers of this period discussing
such issues are rare, contributors to MOP in the 1980s were asked
about their parents' experiences of work in the first half of the twentieth
century, and several reported instances of fathers working stoically
through a variety of nervous conditions. One woman, born in 1915,
explained that her father 'worked as the London salesman of a manufacturing firm in Lancs which was founded by his brother. Although
very successful father hated his work, which resulted in nervous
exhaustion and chronic digestive trouble.'[22] This latter was a very
common proxy for nervous conditions throughout the twentieth century
and, according to Edgar Jones and Simon Wessely, can be seen as part
of a pattern whereby 'particular symptoms appear in specific periods
as a result of underlying cultural trends'.[23] Thus, the symptoms of an
ulcer or suspected ulcer were culturally more acceptable and better
understood at a popular level as indicators of overwork or strain than
more psychological manifestations.[24] This is reflected in the account
of another MOP correspondent born in the 1920s, whose father worked

as Chief Clerk in the local Education Office and suffered with an ulcer so that 'much of his life he was in discomfort and sometimes severe pain. He never spoke about this or theorised as to what was the cause of the illness though the doctor talked a lot about "bottling up emotion" and being "over-conscientious" (this was repeated by mother).'[25] The doctor's comments clearly hint at stress, but such explanations were evidently not acceptable to the father who perhaps viewed them as signs of mental weakness or as inappropriate for someone in his position.

The role of work in everyday life and the way that it was conceptualised played a significant part in how people recognised and understood such experiences and explanations, or why they chose to ignore them. The period in which the IHRB was carrying out its research was one in which many people were simply glad to have any work regardless of its suitability or the impact it might have on their physical or psychological health. The economic recessions of the 1920s and 1930s brought widespread unemployment to many areas of Britain and as research at the time showed, among the long-term unemployed at least a third lived below the poverty line, many of them barely at a subsistence level. Such poverty meant insufficient money to be adequately fed, warm or clothed.[26] When recession struck, employers were most likely to rid themselves of their least productive workers first, and get rid of the roles that had provided employment for the infirm and the elderly, who may have been kept on as a reward for loyalty and long service as much as for any productive capacity they might have.[27] In such circumstances, workers clung to their employment, regardless of any nervous problems, and were highly unlikely to express their suffering, and certainly not in terms that might suggest any sort of medical problem. Even admitting to being a bit 'nervy' or 'highly strung' or suffering with stomach problems might risk their employment.

'Work was "life", without it you did not survive. It came first and last, always waiting to be done.'[28] This was a railwayman's comment to MOP about his work in the 1930s. It illustrates how the necessity of work for survival framed everyday attitudes for most working-class and many lower middle-class families. Similarly, a Police Sergeant recalled his childhood impressions of work in the same period: 'I formed the distinct impression that WORK WAS BLOODY UNENJOYABLE. Owing to my parents having to work hard – long hours ... Work in those days was not secure – and a continual reminder was the WORK-HOUSE situated right at the bottom of the street.'[29] The threat of the workhouse and fear of poverty were powerful motivators to do work of any kind, regardless of its nature and how one felt about it. Moreover, for many people, the relationship with their employer was based on a psychological contract that traded security of employment for loyalty, respect and an acceptance of whatever shortcomings or even hazards accompanied the job. The frequency of unemployment in some regions in the period meant security was *the* priority and this meant many people accepted whatever conditions of work and treatment were forthcoming. An enquiry into happiness carried out in Bolton in the 1930s revealed that economic security was the dominant consideration.[30] For those working or growing up during the decades before the creation of the welfare state, work was an absolute necessity for survival. It could be unpleasant, poorly rewarded and insecure and whether you liked it or not was irrelevant: and if it affected your nerves, you had little choice but to get on with it. In such conditions, even articulating one's feelings of strain or stress in the privacy of home was largely pointless, when to some extent a constant state of anxiety about the risk of unemployment was the norm.

While economic imperatives were the obvious motivation for work, contemporary research into unemployment revealed its role in psychoneurotic illness and anxiety states, as well as the additional latent consequences of employment for human experience that went beyond the economic.[31] Those consequences focused on the significance of work in imposing a daily time structure; shared experiences and contacts outside the family; links to goals and a purpose beyond the individual's own intentions; personal status and identity; and imposed activity.[32] These factors made work psychologically supportive and emphasised the contribution of work to the individual's sense of identity and status, belonging and social life, as well as to the basic economics of survival. However, they also added to the complexities of acknowledging the experience of workplace neurosis.

Work provided status and acknowledged fulfilment of duty to family and society. As a teacher born in 1929 told MOP, 'There is little doubt that my generation were deeply influenced by the Victorian work ethic: to work hard is GOOD; to slack is SINFUL.'[33] Without doubt, there was a moral danger in being workless whether by choice or not. Within this conceptual framework to find work stressful was akin to a dereliction of duty, shameful and a threat to the family, not just the individual. Work was also a fundamental factor in constructing a sense of identity, as another MOP correspondent growing up in the interwar period commented, of her mother, 'To say my mother enjoyed her work would be an understatement. My mother was her work for many, many years, if not the whole of her life.'[34] Her comment is interesting for its emphasis on the importance of work for her mother, as attitudes to work were largely based on a gendered understanding of work as something that happened outside the home and specifically valued men's work. A teacher explained the mindset he was brought up with in the period: 'Work was a bestower of status, in that inside the home the breadwinner was absolute king and certain work had status outside the home.'[35]

Thus, work was a measure of self-worth, particularly for men, acknowledged as the main breadwinners for most of the century. This tied the meaning of work very closely to meanings of masculinity so that it was 'bound up with the labour process, the notion of skills and the experience of work'.[36] A twenty-seven-year-old man commented in a 1937 MO survey that a friend was 'showing distinct signs of nervous strain' largely because of the excessively long hours he worked and because he was 'bullied by his employer'. However, he was opposing any attempts by his wife to return to work so that he could leave and find another less stressful role. The respondent concluded that this was because he saw such a solution as an affront to his 'masculinity'.[37] A machine-tool operator who started work between the wars explained, '35 years I worked in an engineering workshop. It was "mans" work. Hard, dirty and to me, satisfying.'[38] The very hardship of some work in itself became a source of pride, as men reframed their experiences of dangerous, uncomfortable or distressing work in a way which created a masculine virtue of the toughness they needed to endure, but that also fundamentally excluded even the possibility of psychological suffering.[39]

Consequently, the meaning of work mediated the relationship between work and stress. That meaning was constructed around economics, identity and purpose. This meant that work-related experiences which were troubling or damaging to health, whether physical or psychological, could be problematic in multiple ways, as admitting even to oneself that something at work was causing psychological distress threatened poverty, loss of status for individual and family, social life and ultimately even one's sense of existential purpose in the world. Employers might be exploitative, conditions harsh, tasks boring or colleagues difficult, but enduring all of that was the cultural norm.

This disconnect between the experience of the worker and the effect of the work or workplace was simply a case of ignoring a problem which both wished to downplay: workers because they relied on their job for survival and employers because it did not register as their responsibility. If you were ill that was your problem, and in such circumstances, it seems fair to conjecture that many whose work did cause them stress were scarcely able to acknowledge it themselves, or as with the IHRB research, only did so when specifically asked by researchers under conditions of anonymity. The IHRB researchers themselves commented that 'It is not easy to detect these people, for their symptoms may not be expressed in unusual behaviour ... They rarely display their mental state; they believe strongly in the power and importance of self-control, which they exercise consciously in various directions.'[40] The effect therefore of insecure employment and fear of poverty was to supress the expression or even acknowledgement of nervous suffering among most workers.

The stoicism of such workers confounded the IHRB study, leaving the researchers with many unanswered questions regarding the effectiveness of nervous people and the difficulties they faced in adapting to 'the ordinary economic environment'.[41] A report on the IHRB research in the *British Journal of Medical Psychology* concluded that just as some people were physically unfit for certain occupations and were therefore denied them, some were 'temperamentally unsuited for particular conditions, and they should be diverted into occupations suitable for them'. However, it noted that 'Much more work is needed for more definite conclusions.'[42] This additional work presumably included identifying exactly how to recognise such people and conditions, and then the much more problematic issue of how to move them into different work. As the report appeared during the Depression, this latter option was unlikely to be possible, and indeed, precarious employment would make it even more unlikely that workers would facilitate the identification of their nervous suffering for fear of losing their job.

Suburban and urban neuroses

It was the move from urban to suburban location that was apparently at the root of another form of nervous suffering also problematic to acknowledge, that of suburban neurosis. Between 1932 and 1939 local authorities rehoused about four-fifths of those living in slums, and between 1919 and 1939 built 1.5 million dwellings, with most towns and cities gaining large municipal estates. That many of the rehoused were overjoyed at the nature of their new homes was reflected in the frequency of comments such as 'it was just like a palace'.[43] However, the joys of the material experience of the new home were very soon displaced by a new set of challenges relating to location, community, privacy and isolation. As a vicar interviewed as part of a survey carried out in the 1930s on the Watling estate in Hendon, built in 1927 by London County Council, reported, 'The loneliness of the people here in the first months after their removal to Watling is extreme. The women are mostly affected by that desperate loneliness. They feel as if they have moved to the desert.'[44] Illustrating the attitudes of the new arrivals, one woman on another suburban estate reported of her relationship with her new neighbours, 'I keep myself to myself and I don't talk to any of them. I don't know the name of the lady next door and I don't suppose she knows mine.'[45] Encountering the results of such isolation, Dr Stephen Taylor identified a new, psychological complaint, attributable to living on such estates, which he called 'the suburban neurosis' and used to describe the 'young women with anxiety states' presenting at his clinics.

In a *Lancet* article of 1938, Taylor explained that after four years of working in hospital out-patient clinics, he had identified various categories of patient and was sharing his ideas in order to 'throw light' on the environmental causes of neuroses. He described the condition affecting young women, living on the 'wonderful new Everysuburb estate, adjacent to one of our great by-passes and only twenty minutes from the station'.[46] His mocking description captures some of the snobbery that was felt (and continued to be felt throughout the twentieth century) about the suburbs and suburban life, but also the limitations of the middle-class observer trying to understand without disapproval, values and practices he did not share.[47] It was perhaps a way to underpin the existing class boundaries that were threatened by the expansion of cities and improvement of working-class housing stock, or more broadly a way of criticising a very visible part of a more general process of modernisation that dated back to the nineteenth century.[48]

Despite his mocking tone Taylor was serious about the identification of a specific psychological malaise. He drew on his patients' own accounts, including the fact that most denied their own GP's diagnosis of 'nerves', perhaps hoping for a more concrete physical diagnosis. He listed their descriptions of their symptoms, which included 'Trembling all over' and jumping 'at the slightest noise'; 'continuous gnawing, nagging headache'; 'stabbing pains over my heart'; shortness of breath 'when I hurry'; and inability to sleep at night.[49] Manifesting itself in a variety of physical and mental symptoms relating to anxiety states, he suggested the causes were rooted in the environment:

> Few who have not worked or lived in the suburbs can realise the intense loneliness of their unhappy inhabitants. There is no common meeting-ground like the pub and the street of the slum dwellers, and the golf and tennis club of the upper-middle classes. There is no community of interest such as is found in the village. Lack of individual enterprise, shyness and bashfulness prevent calling, and the striking up of friendships. It is respectable to keep oneself to oneself. The Englishman's home is still his castle, but for the Englishwoman too often it is her gaol.[50]

Taylor's observation about respectability and keeping oneself to oneself was an astute one. Poverty had forced the poorest to live their lives in public in the inner cities through the sharing of facilities and reliance on community for support.[51] It was the desire to escape this that provided the key stimulus in persuading people to quit towns and cities for the suburbs.[52] Indeed, privacy was revealed as a major concern in an MO survey in the early 1940s: a woman living in a new block of urban flats complained, 'Everyone should have privacy. We've got a balcony, but the lady next door can see into it', while another woman in similar circumstances explained, 'We have to wash in the scullery and people in the top of the opposite block can look in.'[53] This attitude fuelled a powerful desire to pull up the drawbridge on the Englishman's and Englishwoman's castle: 'Well I'm not complaining. The neighbours here are very nice. But they have their reserve. You might be dead and they wouldn't know.'[54] There was evidently a paradox in the desire for privacy which while highly valued, also involved losing some of the benefits of the community of the slums, as one woman who had moved out of London to new flats described, 'They're not neighbourly here. My husband's out all day. There's nothing going on. As I say, I like a jolly good fight to watch. Mind you, I don't want to be in it. It's all right for young people out at business, they like it quiet when they come home.'[55]

The movement of working-class families from the slums of the cities into suburban housing estates led to higher levels of material comfort, but with this came increased expectations of continuing improvements, focusing on the home as evidence of both social advancement and burgeoning consumerism.[56] This increased materialism helped to blur class boundaries, but such social instability also contributed to a reluctance to make visible any perceived shortcomings. Thus, many of the housewives on the new estates were reluctant to relieve their own unhappiness by approaching neighbours, who in most cases were in very similar situations of isolation themselves, because they feared exposing their own homes to scrutiny in case they did not come up to scratch, both in terms of standards of housework but also quality of material possessions. Being able to keep house more than adequately was integral to the housewife identity and for some women perhaps there was too much at stake to risk damaging that through the imagined criticisms of others. Also at work was the readjustment from the clearly understood working-class context of the slums to a more indefinite class understanding on new housing estates. As late as the 1970s research on suburban life showed the contradictory attitudes of new inhabitants of such estates, some concerned that their new environment was too socially superior, while others found it inferior.[57] While slum living had reduced most inhabitants to the lowest common denominator in terms of class, social status on the new suburban estates was more difficult to quantify, and this contributed to the inhabitants' insecurities. As one explained, 'They should separate the different kinds of people. Our next-door neighbours are common and use very bad language. The rough people should be put together. I don't want to have a lot to do with my neighbours, but I want to *like* them.'[58]

Women newly moved to the suburbs therefore lived with contradictory emotions: they had achieved the longed-for new home and escaped the squalor of the inner city, but paradoxically they felt worse for it. On the one hand, they had wanted the physical benefits of sanitation, space and light, and were very happy with the new housing that provided this, but on the other this came with the fulfilment of a desire for privacy which ultimately revealed that it was not privacy per se that had surely been desired, but the *option* of privacy. Many were used to living in communities sharing basic services such as lavatories and washing facilities and were accustomed to the solidarity of shared deprivation. The new housing gave them greater privacy, but it also meant there were fewer points of contact to maintain or rebuild communal feeling, and once a practice of living more privately became normalised, it created a self-fulfilling cycle which was very difficult to break. That they were also reluctant to accept the diagnosis of 'nerves' from their GPs suggests a desire to supress these contradictory emotions. It would be much easier to admit to some physical problem than to the psychological effects of change.

It was not just the self-imposed loneliness that underpinned suburban neurosis. There was also the increased financial struggle of making ends meet that resulted from higher rents and the cost of travel to work for their husbands. Taylor noted in his discussion of causation that anxiety about 'money and house' was justifiable due to the financial commitments of suburban living and the risks that might arise if the breadwinner became ill.[59] He also noted that lack of friends was a key issue, but whereas men's social needs were largely met in the workplace, the increased travel time and reduced available money meant husbands were often too tired, unwilling or unable on returning home in the evening to meet the social needs of their lonely wives, often revealing the previously hidden limitations of some marriages. In many instances, the opportunities for local leisure or social activities were limited, if not non-existent, as the estates had no shops or pubs that might provide a focus for socialising. One woman from an estate responding to an MO survey about housing commented, 'Well, there's no life.'[60] While the new housing might be clean compared to the slums, for many, the estates seemed soulless: 'I don't like these endless roads – there is no variety in the district at present', was another woman's comment, while a Cockney ex-slum dweller stated, 'I dislike everything. I'd sooner be back in London. I don't like the country.'[61]

According to Taylor it was not simply the environment of the new housing estates that was to blame, however. It was also the women themselves. He argued that for these newly suburban women it was their inadequacies of mind, false values that fetishised the home and consumption, and disappointment with a husband who 'turns out to be rather ordinary and grumpy' that also played an important part.[62] He claimed that 'The small labour-saving house, the small family, and the few friends have left the women of the suburbs relatively idle. They have nothing to look forward to, nothing to look up to and little to live for.'[63] While it has since been argued that there was little basis for Taylor's image of a bored and leisured housewife, the uptake of labour-saving devices, for example, being extremely small in the period and Taylor's construction of suburban neurosis based partly on conflicting positions in psychiatry and partly in his own patrician suspicion of mass culture, evidently the women living in the new estates were suffering from something that affected their nerves.[64] Whether it was the location of their homes, the limitations of their social interactions or their own inadequacies that were the causes, Taylor's diagnosis of a psychological problem apparently specific to suburban housewives would inform ideas about suburban living for a further forty years.

Taylor's proposed solution in the 1930s was somewhat unrealistic, involving the establishment on each new estate of a team of psycho-analysts to treat the inhabitants. He also suggested that the neurotic housewives would find 'A carefully graded reading list' to be more use 'than a bottle of medicine', revealing snobbery rather than pragmatism, and argued that 'We have allowed the slum which stunted the body to be replaced by a slum which stunts the mind.'[65] His most practical advice was that new estates should establish 'social non-religious clubs catering for all possible interests … something not unlike the Pioneer Health Centre at Peckham.'[66] This was an interesting recommendation as the Peckham project operated in an undoubtedly *urban* context, far from the suburban estates that concerned Taylor. However, he was right in identifying a connection, as the researchers at Peckham had also pinpointed the stultifying effects of domestic life on the poor and tackled them from a social as well as medical perspective. Here was an apparent paradox: Taylor had identified the suburbs as causing neurosis, but apparently so could an urban environment. What the two had in common was the apparent importance of interaction with the outside world beyond the home, and the gendered nature of domestic stress. Evidently, there was something at work in the domestic environment which caused some women to suffer, but Taylor's causative assumption about the geography of the suburbs was too limited an explanation, however popular it might prove with researchers in the coming decades.

The Pioneer Health Centre in Peckham

The Pioneer Health Centre (PHC) in Peckham was set up by two doctors, George Williamson and Innes Pearse, as a research experiment to test their ideas about health and the necessary conditions for its maintenance. As such, its focus was on identifying the factors that promoted positive health, rather than simply on treating ill-health. Operating intermittently between 1926 and 1950, it functioned as a club for families who agreed to submit to regular medical examinations, and in return were offered a range of services including a crèche, sports facilities and the sale of fresh produce from a farm in Kent.[67] The researchers at Peckham studied both physical illness and psychological well-being and revealed the deadening effects of domestic life:

> The young urban family builds through no fault of its own, not a rich protean body – a *home* that grows out from the nucleus of parenthood, but a poor hovel of sleeping and eating, breeding and clothing. For all too often the family holds no converse with the outside world; its functional scope is restricted to its own hearth and there is little to sustain and feed its members but what happens within the four walls of the house.[68]

They uncovered a greater level of 'disease, disorder and deficiency' in women between the ages of twenty to forty-five than in men and concluded that men's work outside the home, though often unfulfilling and leaving little leisure, did provide a level of stimulation and external interaction that staved off 'stagnation': a finding that echoed the contemporary research on unemployment and the latent consequences of work, discussed earlier in this chapter.[69] However, for women, they concluded, it was different: 'Marriage is apt to lead her into conditions in which social stagnation and inaction are almost unavoidable.'[70] In their view, a wide range of problems, both medical and social, arose from the domestic norm of such families, including 'every form of chronic and acute disease and disorder in the home; disharmony, neurasthenia, inebriety, "suburban neurosis", causes for divorce, parental neglect or incompetence, the difficult child, the young offender; suspicion, retreat and anti-social behaviour of all sorts'. These were the result of the 'functional starvation' of people living in physical structures that were not really homes.[71]

The 1943 book about the first two phases of the project, *The Peckham Experiment: A Study in the Living Structure of Society*, described one such couple, Mr and Mrs X, married for seven years with two children aged four and two whom the wife was 'incapable of managing'. She was described as 'fat, flabby, constipated, dressed in slovenly clothes' and 'was suspicious, diffident and negative. The husband was overweight, irritable with his wife in private, in public alternating between over-confidence and shyness.'[72] This unfortunate couple were 'disillusioned; life to them had become stagnant, if not sour', with the husband rising at six o'clock for work and his wife remaining in bed until nine or later and giving the children their breakfast at ten o'clock, and then, as the book described:

> She cooked a desultory dinner of one course; walked up and down the shopping street three or four afternoons a week with the baby strapped into the pram, the elder child dragging beside her; went to the park once a week, speaking to no one and coming home early because the elder child was fretful: knew no one except for a passing acquaintance with the grocer's wife round the corner, and her in-laws, with whom she was on the defensive and did not find herself in sympathy.[73]

Another couple of slightly better social status and with only one child, whose case was also recounted, were described as 'diffident', and so irritable and critical with each other and the child that it was apparent to the researchers at their first meeting that the wife was 'not far off a nervous breakdown'. The PHC researchers reported that 'these are not pictures of families standing out vividly by reason of their rarity. Varying but slightly in detail, this story of early married life is repeated with *monotonous regularity*.'[74]

Their answer was to provide medical solutions to physical ills and to address psychological problems via a wide range of social opportunities for both women and men through the PHC. For the unfortunate Mr and Mrs X, this meant a referral to a gynaecologist for her as well as taking up keep-fit classes, dress-making and badminton, while he joined the boxing club and started teaching boxing to boys as well as playing badminton with his wife. Eventually they 'built up a social circle of their own, coming out perhaps two evenings a week'. Such activities led to both losing weight, moving about 'more briskly' and looking healthier. The reported effects on their children included cessation of bed-wetting, weight gain and better socialisation. For the other couple, discussing their problems at the PHC and a gradual increase in social activities led to greater confidence so that the husband gained a promotion and his wife 'became an educative force with the other mothers'.[75] From the researchers' point of view, a home only really functioned as such when its occupants also had external interests and social interaction with the outside world. Without these, instead of being a source of comfort and safety, it was one of tension and misery. Unfortunately, this was at odds with the aspirations of many of the poorest, working-class women who, after years of sharing facilities under the scrutiny of others, were focused on *not* interacting with others and being able to close the door on the world.[76]

The PHC researchers believed that health was not simply the absence of illness, but that promoting and maintaining it required a different approach to curing disease. This change of perspective reflected a shift from seeing illness as the normal state of being to a more optimistic stance that viewed health as the norm. Their approach emphasised the 'organic and the whole, rather than medicine', and built on their view that good health arose from the relationship between the human organism and its environment with the family as the 'fundamental unit of society'.[77] Thus both the PHC researchers and Taylor were making a fundamentally similar argument: family and home were not sufficient in themselves for good mental health. Instead, it was the juxtaposition of home and the outside world fuelled by interactions with others that made life meaningful and enabled people to live healthily. The home only functioned as a haven if there was something to retreat from, otherwise, as Taylor implied, it was potentially a gaol and the cause of unhappiness and neurosis to its occupants.

During the 1920s and 1930s, while some research focused specifically on finding neurosis and its sufferers in a work context, driven by concerns about productivity, other researchers encountered a domestic version as part of a wider concern about the health of the urban and suburban poor. In both cases, such experiences were problematised not by the sufferers but by those interested in him or her as either worker or inhabitant of a particular location. Although much of the research into nervous suffering in both a work and domestic context was focused on the environment as a cause, at the heart of most explanations was a belief in the inherent weakness of the individual in failing to adequately adapt to their environment.

Conclusion

While the language of researchers and doctors mostly focused on neurosis to describe the experience of their subjects in this period, the people themselves talked about their nerves, of being highly strung and of nervous breakdown, if they talked about them at all. Within the various experiences so described was a vast range of different symptoms and conditions as the IHRB researchers acknowledged. Thus, some of what they were describing might fit within our contemporary notion of stress, while other elements, as Taylor suggested in his explanation of suburban neurosis, might be closer to depression.[78] However, what matters is that such experiences were being singled out as the focus of an organisational and medical discourse that framed them as problematic. The IHRB was interested in identifying workers with 'neurotic tendencies' as part of a much larger context of scientific management that was keen to quantify all manner of aspects of work, with a particular focus on ways of improving productivity and categorising workers. While its research did manage to identify neurotic workers, it proved difficult to draw concrete conclusions because of the inconsistency of worker experience: some people seemed to be able to work effectively despite their suffering while others could not. This was partly due to the very complex nature of people's relationship with work. Workers accepted their conditions of work in return for security, practising a stoicism that meant that you worked on, regardless of what effects your work might have on you, physical or mental. The economic necessity of work for survival framed everyday attitudes, while work was also bound up with critical elements of human experience such as gender identity, status and social needs. This meant that anything that threatened work, such as stressful experiences, also threatened survival and those other factors. This made them problematic to acknowledge and so sufferers used a lay language of nerves (highly strung and/or nervy), the imprecision of which often underplayed the condition while also incorporating a wide range of actual experiences and symptoms. Where people did acknowledge their nervous suffering, it was often via physical symptoms that were a more acceptable and comprehensible expression of strain and mental distress than any psychological explanation. Often such symptoms related to stomach complaints or ulcers which for much of the century were particularly associated with stress both in medical and popular understandings.

Similarly unacknowledgeable, was the fact that although a home might function as a retreat from the world, it might also prove a source of neurosis, particularly for women. Concerns about the health of the poorest classes of society were the basis for the work of the researchers in Peckham but soon revealed that as well as physical illness, there was also a level of mental distress particularly associated with their urban housing environment. This was mirrored by Taylor's identification of a similar mental condition, 'suburban neurosis', amongst those who had escaped urban poverty for the supposedly happier environs of the suburbs but found it wanting. In both cases, the distress that was observed resulted from a lack of interaction with the outside world often underpinned by a privileging of privacy that resulted in a vicious circle of loneliness, isolation and boredom. Certainly, the domestic experience of the women studied reinforced the findings of contemporary work on unemployment which emphasised the importance of work outside the home in providing structure, purpose and social interaction. However, although such ideas were emerging during the 1930s, many of them seemed to be forgotten when war broke out and both government and organisations were faced with the joint problem of motivating conscripted workers and dealing with the dual domestic and employed role that large numbers of women found themselves facing. The behaviour of British workers would be critical to the outcome of the war, yet considerations of the effects of the daily challenges of wartime living did not feature in the government's initial considerations about the psychological effects of war.

Notes

1 Millais Culpin and May Smith, 'The Nervous Temperament: Medical Research Council Report 61' (London: Industrial Health Research Board, 1930), p. iii.

2 *Ibid.*

3 *Ibid.*

4 Taylor, 'Suburban Neurosis', p. 759.

5 Innes H. Pearse and Lucy H. Crocker, *The Peckham Experiment: A Study in the Living Structure of Society* (London: George Allen and Unwin Ltd, 1943).

6 Frederick Winslow Taylor, *The Principles of Scientific Management* (New York; London: Harper, 1911).

7 Elton Mayo, *The Human Problems of Industrial Civilisation* (New York: Macmillan, 1933).

8 Arthur McIvor, 'Employers, the Government, and Industrial Fatigue in Britain, 1890–1918', *British Journal of Industrial Medicine* 44, 11 (November 1987): p. 731.

9 Melling, 'Workplace Fear', p. 201.

10 Ronnie Johnston and Arthur McIvor, 'Marginalising the Body at Work? Employers' Occupational Health Strategies and Occupational Medicine in Scotland c. 1930–1974', *Social History of Medicine* 21, 1 (2008): p. 132, https://doi.org/10.1093/shm/hkn003.

11 *Ibid.*, p. 133.

12 *Ibid.*, p. 137.

13 Melling, 'Labouring Stress', p. 167.

14 Culpin and Smith, 'Nervous Temperament', p. iii.

15 *Ibid.*, pp. 2, 7.

16 *Ibid.*, pp. 9–10.

17 *Ibid.*, p. 12.

18 *Ibid.*, p. 10.

19 Thomson, 'Neurasthenia', pp. 82–7.

20 Culpin and Smith, 'Nervous Temperament', pp. 27, 30.

21 *Ibid.*

22 'Replies to Summer Directive Work' (1983), MOA, University of Sussex, A008.

23 Edgar Jones and Simon Wessely, 'War Syndromes: The Impact of Culture on Medically Unexplained Symptoms', *Medical History* 49, 1 (2005): p. 56, https://doi.org/10.1017/S0025727300008280.

24 Jones, 'Gut War', p. 43.

25 MOA 'Work', A008.

26 Richard Smith, '"Please Never Let It Happen Again": Lessons on Unemployment from the 1930s', *BMJ* 291, 26 October (1985): p. 1191.

27 Noel Whiteside, 'Counting the Cost – Sickness and Disability among Working People in the Era of Industrial Recession, 1920–39', *Economic History Review* 40, 2 (May 1987): p. 240.

28 MOA 'Work', A005.
29 MOA 'Work', R461. Although the 1929 Local Government Act effectively abolished workhouses, local authorities assumed responsibility for such institutions and many were still housing people at the end of the 1930s; see Margaret Anne Crowther, *The Workhouse System, 1834–1929: The History of an English Social Institution* (London: Batsford Academic and Educational, 1981), p. 110.
30 Ian Gazeley and Claire Langhamer, 'The Meanings of Happiness in Mass Observation's Bolton', *History Workshop Journal* 1, 75 (2012): pp. 161–2, 182, https://doi.org/10.1093/hwj/dbs015.
31 For example, James L. Halliday, 'Psychoneurosis as a Cause of Incapacity among Insured Persons', *BMJ* 1 supplement 1584, 3870, 9 March (1935), https://doi.org/10.1136/bmj.1.3870.S85; Philip Eisenberg and Paul F. Lazarsfeld, 'The Psychological Effects of Unemployment', *Psychological Bulletin* 35 (1938): p. 378, http://dx.doi.org/10.1037/h0063426. Research identified the so-called stage theories of unemployment, which, although since challenged on the grounds of methodology, provide insight into the meaning of work relevant to the relationship between work and stress. For an overview, see Marie Jahoda, 'Work, Employment, and Unemployment: Values, Theories, and Approaches in Social Research', *American Psychologist* 36, 2 (1981): p. 189, https://doi.org/10.1037/0003-066x. 36.2.184.
32 *Ibid.*, p. 189.
33 MOA 'Work', A008.
34 MOA 'Work', H675.
35 MOA 'Work', M361.
36 Steven Maynard, 'Rough Work and Rugged Men: The Social Construction of Masculinity in Working-Class History', *Labour / Le Travail* 23, Spring (1989): p. 159, https://doi.org/10.2307/25143139.
37 'Replies to Day Survey, 12th May' (1937), MOA, University of Sussex, 512.
38 MOA 'Work', L689.
39 Nick Hayes, 'Did Manual Workers Want Industrial Welfare? Canteens, Latrines and Masculinity on British Building Sites 1918–1970', *Journal of Social History* 35, 3 (2002): p. 640, https://doi.org/jstor.org/stable/3790694; Paul Willis, 'Shop-Floor Culture, Masculinity and the Wage Form', in John Clarke, C. Critcher and Richard Johnson (eds) *Working-Class Culture: Studies in History and Theory* (London: Hutchinson & Co. Ltd, 1979), p. 196.
40 Culpin and Smith, 'Nervous Temperament', p. 10.
41 *Ibid.*, pp. 27, 30.

42 May Smith, 'The Nervous Temperament', *British Journal of Medical Psychology* 10, 2 (1 June 1930): p. 174, https://doi.org/10.1111/j.2044-8341.1930.tb01014.x.

43 Mark Clapson, *Invincible Green Suburbs, Brave New Towns: Social Change and Urban Dispersal in Postwar England* (Manchester: Manchester University Press, 1998), pp. 33–4.

44 Ruth Durant, *Watling: A Survey of Social Life on a New Housing Estate* (London: P. S. King & Son, 1939), p. 60.

45 *An Enquiry into People's Homes: A Report Prepared by Mass Observation for the Advertising Service Guild* (London: John Murray, 1943), p. 206.

46 Taylor, 'Suburban Neurosis', p. 759.

47 Mark Clapson, 'Working-Class Women's Experiences of Moving to New Housing Estates in England since 1919', *Twentieth Century British History* 10, 3 (1 January 1999): p. 347, https://doi.org/10.1093/tcbh/10.3.345.

48 Judy Giles, *The Parlour and the Suburb: Domestic Identities, Class, Femininity and Modernity* (Oxford: Berg, 2004), pp. 29–30.

49 Taylor, 'Suburban Neurosis', p. 759.

50 *Ibid.*, p. 760.

51 Melanie Tebbutt, *Women's Talk? A Social History of 'Gossip' in Working-Class Neighbourhoods, 1880–1960* (Aldershot: Scolar Press, 1995), p. 88.

52 Clapson, *Suburbs*, p. 133.

53 *People's Homes*, p. 172.

54 *Ibid.*, pp. 206–7.

55 *Ibid.*, p. 198.

56 Clapson, *Suburbs*, p. 98.

57 Bernard Ineichen, 'Neurotic Wives in a Modern Residential Suburb: A Sociological Profile', *Social Science & Medicine* 9, 8–9 (1975): p. 485, https://doi.org/10.1016/0037-7856(75)90077-3.

58 *People's Homes*, p. 207. Italics in the original.

59 Taylor, 'Suburban Neurosis', p. 760.

60 *People's Homes*, p. 198.

61 *Ibid.*, pp. 199, 190.

62 Taylor, 'Suburban Neurosis', pp. 760–1.

63 *Ibid.*, p. 761.

64 Hayward, 'Desperate Housewives', pp. 51, 56.

65 Taylor, 'Suburban Neurosis', p. 761.

66 *Ibid.*

67 Jane Lewis and Barbara Brookes, 'A Reassessment of the Work of the Peckham Health Centre, 1926–1951', *Milbank Memorial Fund Quarterly: Health and Society* 61, 2 (1983): p. 307, https://doi.org/10.2307/3349909.

68 Pearse and Crocker, *Peckham Experiment*, p. 248. Italics in the original.
69 *Ibid.*, p. 254. Eisenberg and Lazarsfeld, 'Psychological Effects', p. 358.
70 Pearse and Crocker, *Peckham Experiment*, p. 254.
71 *Ibid.*, pp. 250–1.
72 *Ibid.*, pp. 249–50.
73 *Ibid.*, p. 250.
74 *Ibid.*, p. 253, p. 251.
75 *Ibid.*, pp. 251–3. Italics in the original.
76 Judy Giles, 'A Home of One's Own: Women and Domesticity in England 1918–1950', *Women's Studies International Forum* 16, 3 (1993): p. 243, https://doi.org/10.1016/0277-5395(93)90054-d.
77 Lewis and Brookes, 'Peckham Health Centre', pp. 308, 313.
78 Taylor mentions that some symptoms appear, like melancholia. Taylor, 'Suburban Neurosis', p. 761.

3

'Just Nerves!': civilian nerves in the Second World War

'It's not the bombs I'm scared of any more, it's the weariness ... trying to work and concentrate with your eyes sticking out of your head like hat-pins, after being up all night. I'd die in my sleep, happily, if only I *could* sleep.'[1] This was the complaint of a female civil servant in the early days of the London Blitz, her comment reflecting the way civilian responses to war on the Home Front during the Second World War were often characterised by stoicism and even humour.[2] Such framing of people's experiences occurred both retrospectively in nostalgic accounts of a Blitz spirit, but also at the time by the wartime coalition government keen to confirm that the psychological impact of air raids was far less than had been anticipated before the war. Indeed, fears of aerial warfare in the 1930s had led to considerable alarm about potential civilian casualties, both physical and psychiatric, and a 'blood-curdling picture' of what would happen if London were bombed.[3] Chamberlain's pre-war government, therefore, prepared for large-scale casualties, anticipating psychiatric cases would outnumber the physical by three to one.[4] In the event, such pessimism proved unfounded. Only 5 per cent of all air-raid casualties were found to suffer from nervous shock, most recovering within a fortnight, and by December 1940 admissions to special psychiatric hospitals numbered only twenty-five in London and three in the whole of the rest of England. As a result, these facilities were stood down and it was generally understood that Britons had turned out to be more psychologically resilient to war than expected; a conclusion that sat comfortably within the 'Britain can take it' position of wartime propaganda.[5]

However, in July 1941 Tom Harrisson, one of the co-founders of the MO research organisation, and now working on commission for the Ministry of Information, carrying out a range of wartime research on topics such as morale, told a meeting of the British Psychological Society that although the limited number of psychiatric casualties arising from air raids so far was 'cheering and encouraging', it did not give 'the whole of the picture'. Harrisson claimed that the 'mass of ordinary, normal people who do not react to raids with definite neurotic or hysterical symptoms such as demand individual clinical treatment' was nevertheless 'very profoundly affected in a number of ways', which would not come to the attention of a practising psychologist.[6] Part of his concern was the effect of bombing on towns and cities outside of London, where their size and more limited resources meant that the impact of the loss of loved ones, homes, services and the familiar landmarks of everyday life was more devastating, particularly in the absence of strong and effective post-raid organisation and leadership. This absence meant that feelings of helplessness and an inability to cope were unnecessarily aggravated and risked seriously intensifying 'harmful psychological tendencies'.[7]

Harrisson's concern that the bombing was having a greater psychological impact than the government acknowledged was supported by MO research carried out earlier in 1941 on the psychological effects of air raids. This had shown that despite 'neurotic tendencies' being the 'exception rather than the rule', approximately half of MO informants had come across occasional cases and thus 'we cannot accept the widely-held opinion that raids have not led to any nervous breakdown'.[8] Indeed, the Ministry of Home Security carried out a survey on the psychological after-effects of air raids and sent a team of psychiatrists to Hull which had experienced a series of heavy raids in the spring and summer of 1941. Many of those bombed in Hull had persisted in 'trekking' out of the city every night to seek shelter and safety away from the bombs and this was taken to suggest they had been more badly affected by the raids. The wartime government's interest was not particularly in their psychological well-being, but on whether bombing caused psychological collapse, which might provoke social breakdown.[9] Although the researchers did find that some men and women remained seriously neurotic six months after the bombings, and others suffered from moderate or slight neurosis, they reported that more than half of the sample researched appeared to have no symptoms at all. This was sufficient for them to conclude that there was no particularly high incidence of neurosis, or bad morale in Hull.[10] Nevertheless, as Overy has pointed out, a high proportion of the Hull inhabitants who were interviewed had case sheets showing symptoms that were far from normal, such as vomiting at the sound of a siren, fainting, crying, depression, insomnia and severe dyspepsia.[11]

The reality of the psychological impact of aerial bombardment lay somewhere between the official view of a psychologically unscathed population and the experience of MO's on-the-ground investigators who saw with their own eyes the effects on people caught up in raids. Their reports included examples such as one middle-aged woman who explained, 'after having my husband blown out of bed … when I hear the sirens now I'm all like this … (hands shaking). But we've got to keep ourselves in hand haven't we? The doctor said to me afterwards, it's no use you being like this. But it makes you nervous, after you've been bombed once and blown out of bed.'[12] In many cases, such people simply did not appear in official statistics because they did not present at hospitals, and with the emphasis after raids being on physical clear up, people were simply left to recover as best they could.[13]

Of course, people *were* anxious and afraid of air raids and many did not share in the Blitz spirit that became the popular perception of wartime life in the decades after the war.[14] However, in those towns and cities, particularly London, which experienced the most prolonged and extensive blitz, they mostly adjusted to the wartime way of life, including its many anxieties, and effectively became accustomed to living with such underlying strain. Indeed, analysis of post-blitz morale by the Air Ministry suggested that the frequency of raids effectively 'conditioned' people to bombing, enabling them to cope better.[15] This was also consistent with the expectations of good wartime citizenship, which depended on 'stoical acceptance of suffering' and an emotional economy of reticence and restraint, whether dealing with grief, fear or other emotions thrown up by wartime experiences.[16] It was also because, for most, there was little else they could do, and thus a combination of fatalism, stoicism and resignation was as much a characteristic of wartime behaviour as the cheery resolve mythologised as the spirit of the Blitz both during and after the war. For it was not necessarily the strain of living with air raids that took the greatest toll on the mental well-being of most civilian Britons, but the more wearisome exigencies of everyday wartime life.

This chapter examines the experience of wartime stress, focusing not on the extremes of psychiatric damage originally envisaged by Chamberlain's pre-war Government, but on the long-term, mundane strain of day-to-day life on the Home Front. It reveals a more complex picture of wartime life that both contradicts and upholds ideas of Britons as stoically and cheerfully surviving wartime privations, frustrations and destruction. It focuses on wartime workers and the ways in which the challenges of everyday life during the war intersected with the specific demands made of them in a wartime economy. While government concerns were focused particularly on problems of industrial absenteeism and motivation, missed production targets and labour shortages, many of these problems resulted directly from the daily strain of wartime living, as much as issues in the workplace. Several in-depth reports, individual diaries and surveys by MO reveal the day-to-day tensions and problems of organisations contending with a largely conscripted, and sometimes unwilling, workforce. These imply that the long working hours, often monotonous and meaningless tasks, as well as the challenges of local transport, were at the heart of the work-related stress that manifested itself in a level of sickness absence that so concerned the country's leaders.

Compounding the strain on many women workers were the specifically gendered contributions of shopping, rationing and housework. That there was such strain was acknowledged by the publication of a government public health information leaflet in 1943 entitled 'Just Nerves!'[17] Examination of this document offers insight into official views and advice about wartime mental health, while also reconfirming existing ideas about causation and the association of physical and psychological suffering. Its somewhat mixed messages illustrate the limitations on the government's ability to tackle the issue, and its reliance on the good citizenship characteristics of stoicism and selflessness place it squarely within the propagandist messages of the 'People's War'.

Government attempts to tackle issues of absenteeism and under-production included the introduction of more structured welfare services in factories. Reports submitted by Miss Richmond, a Welfare Officer working for a London company, during and just after the war, demonstrate the practical realities of such interventions, and their limitations. Her accounts also illustrate popular attitudes towards those suffering from nerves and nervous breakdown, which largely positioned the sufferer's own weakness at the heart of their nervous suffering.

The final section of the chapter explores a unique organisational attempt to deal with industrial neurosis through the creation of a centre for rehabilitating workers at Roffey Park, set up in 1943 by a group of companies under the auspices of St Thomas' Hospital in London and the National Council for the Rehabilitation of Industrial Workers (NCRIW) and dedicated to treating and returning to productive work those employees who were suffering because of their work. Roffey Park showed what was possible in terms of dealing with such workers but was largely contingent on its specific wartime circumstances and ultimately short-lived, disappearing into general psychiatric provision in the new National Health Service (NHS) after the war.

Overall this chapter suggests that during the Second World War it was the long-term, often mundane strain of everyday life on the Home Front, manifested through absenteeism, or in more extreme cases presented as industrial neurosis or nervous breakdown, that became the focus of governmental and institutional concern about stress, rather than the psychological effects of bombing. It presents a picture of everyday life that is inconsistent with mythologised ideas of uncomplaining stoicism and Blitz spirit and instead suggests a more mundane existence of boredom, frustration and hard slog. While the British government had expected to have to deal with high levels of serious psychiatric casualties resulting from aerial warfare, what they got was a population which, while largely coping with the war, was nevertheless affected by the stress of doing so. Yet wartime circumstances made it harder for people to acknowledge and articulate their nervous suffering because not only were many people in similar situations, it was also evident that others at home and overseas were exposed to much greater physical danger and horrifying experiences. It was also inconsistent with the propagandist rhetoric of perseverance that required people to uphold communal morale. Therefore, in those cases where individuals were no longer able to cope, this was largely understood as an inherent weakness of the individual, particularly within this context of expected collective wartime stoicism.

Nervy civilians

'I think it's mostly the strain. I think everybody's worried and nervy these days.' This was the response of a thirty-five-year-old woman to an MO survey about health in 1943. While most people felt their health had suffered because of the war, the reasons given were somewhat vague. As another woman explained, 'It seems as if war undermines one's whole physique. I can't make out whether it's the strain on the nerves, different feeding, lack of sleep or suggestion', while another added, 'Too much work and worry.' The author of the survey report concluded that 'It is not clear whether references to nerves show that these are the real cause, or whether poor health is the cause of bad nerves, but certainly the two are intertwined in some way.'[18] The idea that 'suggestion' might be involved in creating neurosis was linked particularly to concerns about patent medicine advertisements and as early as August 1940 MO had investigated whether commercial advertisers were using the fears and attendant problems of air raids to publicise their goods.[19] Although they concluded that this was not the case, nevertheless manufacturers of a range of products from Cadbury's Bourn-vita drink to patent medicines such as Yeast-Vite tablets and Dr Williams Pink Pills certainly were advertising the supposed restorative effects of their products on wartime nerves as a specific selling point, even if they were not highlighting air raids in particular.[20]

The recognition by commercial organisations of a ready market for products addressing a wide-ranging and vague list of symptoms, including poor sleep, depression, irritability and worry, was not lost on the authorities, who were aware of the constant strain on people of conscription, rationing, long work hours and sleep deprivation. One result was the issue of a leaflet entitled 'Just Nerves!' by the Central Council for Health Education (CCHE), which ran several health education campaigns on topics, including diphtheria inoculation, venereal disease and worker welfare for the Ministry of Health during the war. Distributed via local authorities, educational services and in some cases directly to factories, CCHE literature targeted a wide range of people and at the height of one campaign produced as many as 400,000 leaflets a month.[21] 'Just Nerves!' was a simple twofold A4 leaflet apparently intended to reassure those who were suffering with their 'nerves' and encourage them to seek help, although this empathetic message was somewhat undermined by the closing paragraph's reminder that 'A great many people are in the same boat with you and yet are pulling their weight. And so must you.'[22] Written in plain language with a brisk, practical tone that offered both empathy and a pointed reminder to the reader of their personal responsibilities, it reflected the approach of many of the self-help books discussed in Chapter 1, although it differed in advising sufferers to consult their doctor.

The leaflet set out to normalise people's anxieties – 'We are all inclined to be over-anxious and nervy at times, and perhaps more than ever under the stress of present-day conditions' – while also warning against taking 'a special pride in being "nervous" and "sensitive"', or using nerves 'as an excuse for avoiding unpleasant duties or as a weapon to force your family to let you have your own way'. The leaflet offered a broad description of potential symptoms and behaviours: 'things get on your nerves, you become on edge and unhappy; you worry too much over disappointments, slights and lost opportunities; and you begin to feel that nothing goes right with you and that things and people are against you'. It went on to state that, as a result, 'You may lose interest in your usual hobbies, and your anxiety may exhaust you so that you find everything is a trouble and nothing seems worth-while. By the time your work is over you are too tired to enjoy your leisure; and yet you may not be able to sleep properly, but waken in the middle of the night in a cold sweat of anxiety.' This might lead the sufferer to '"worry yourself sick" and develop such things as vague aches and pains, palpitations, stomach trouble and faint turns'. All of this, it hastened to add, was nothing to be ashamed of and did not mean that the sufferer was 'gradually going off your head'. Echoing similar reassurances seen in self-help books and discussed in Chapter 1, this again underlines the very real popular fear that any psychological wobble was the harbinger of full-blown madness.

Against that backdrop, the leaflet unsurprisingly acknowledged that most people would wish to keep their fears and worries to themselves, but went on to equate such mental suffering to physical ills and recommended that as for 'chest trouble, or toothache' the reader seek proper advice from a doctor, suggesting that there might be a physical cause for their nerves such as 'bad teeth'. This may partly have been in keeping with the popular preference for physical explanations over psychological ones, but also a way of encouraging people to seek help for nervous problems while they were still minor in order to avoid serious breakdowns that were bad for general morale. In the absence of a physical cause the leaflet explained that the doctor might refer the reader to a 'clinic where a special study of these problems is made'. It explained that the number of such places was increasing as the need to help people with 'nervous trouble' was being 'more fully recognised'.[23] Such advice was surprising, partly in recognising the potential extent of psychological suffering being caused by wartime conditions, but also in suggesting that there was adequate provision to deal with it. As will be apparent later in the chapter, places such as Roffey Park Rehabilitation Centre, set up to treat industrial neurosis, were the exception rather than the norm and one of the reasons that the Beveridge Report's proposal of a national health service in 1942 was so widely supported was recognition of the woefully inadequate state of all medical provision, not just psychiatry, both before and during the war.[24]

Having suggested recourse to others for help, the leaflet then emphasised the importance of self-help, encouraging the reader to 'deliberately try to think of pleasant and happy things and thus rid your mind of wearing anxiety'. It also recommended sharing worries with 'a sympathetic friend or a person whom you can trust, such as the work's nurse', the latter counsel somewhat optimistically supposing that such a person was available. It ended with a reminder that acts of great bravery were often performed by 'men and women who were terribly afraid' and that 'nerves are a common complaint' and would probably soon be over.[25]

On the one hand, 'Just Nerves!' appeared to reassure people by normalising the stress and anxiety that were undoubtedly a common experience in wartime Britain: a stance that was consistent with wartime propaganda and efforts to maintain morale. It was also encouraging a greater openness about psychological suffering than had previously been the norm, emphasising that there was 'nothing to be ashamed of', and perhaps attempting to harness the power of collective experience, both as a support mechanism, but also as a reminder that everyone was in the same boat. This approach reflected the needs of wartime Britain and the maintenance of a hard-working and resilient population, more than a significant shift in popular attitudes to mental health problems. Indeed, it was also evidently aiming to counter the problem of people shirking responsibilities and using a 'nervous' or 'sensitive' identity to avoid 'unpleasant duties'. Thus, it trod a fine line between a tone of sympathy and exhorting sufferers to pull their weight. Its focus on encouraging readers to see a doctor to determine whether there was a physical cause for their nerves clearly fitted with the common preference for physical explanations for mental distress. Underlying the whole leaflet was the encouragement to keep busy: 'most people find that it helps to have some definite job to do at such times', to accept responsibilities and to do one's duty. It effectively called on individuals to be stoic but also emphasised their role in the collective endeavour. Thus, nerves were both normal and something to take professional advice on if necessary but should otherwise be endured and not allowed to interfere with the demands of wartime life.

Wartime work and well-being

From the state's perspective, this was of paramount importance, not only in terms of morale and stoicism but in very practical ways in terms of people's participation in voluntary service and war work. Until 1941, men between the ages of 20 and 45 were eligible for conscription, with some in so-called 'reserved' occupations exempt from military service. However, this very soon proved insufficient for both military and industrial needs and the age of conscription was lowered to 18 and extended to 51 and reserved occupations effectively abolished, with deferment for key workers granted on a case-by-case basis. In the same year, the government introduced female conscription and by the middle of the war men and women aged 18–60 were required to undertake some form of national service.[26] This might be part or full-time work and/or voluntary civil defence and other war-related duties.[27] While this fulfilled some of the government's manpower requirements, the conscription of workers brought its own problems for employer and worker alike. The efficiency and productivity of industry were critical to the war effort on every front, yet there were continual worker shortages, missed production targets and high levels of absenteeism.

Prompted by concerns about industry and, in particular the prime minister's reference to the crisis of manpower, between October 1941 and April 1942 MO carried out research into industrial efficiency.[28] Published in 1942, and based on conversations with 1,200 workers in eighty firms including contributions from trade union officials, supervisors, managing directors and voluntary observers, *An Enquiry into British War Production – A Report Prepared by Mass Observation for the Advertising Service Guild: Part 1: People in Production* provided considerable insight into the issue of worker well-being, morale and the thorny issue of productivity. In doing so, the *Enquiry* also shed light on some of the more mundane daily struggles that contributed to wartime stress and ultimately worker demotivation.[29] The authors were critical of the status quo: 'In view of its evident importance to production, the extent to which industries and unions concern themselves with the health of their workers is noticeably slight', and their findings linked the welfare and psychological well-being of workers under considerable strain to both motivation and output.[30]

How workers felt about the work they were doing had not initially figured in the government's plans to get everyone working in the wartime economy. Anyone not already doing essential work might be asked to consider one or two jobs that were more important to the war effort and most were willing to conform, but where they were not, they could be compelled into a role, and between July 1941 and June 1942, for example, 32,000 compulsory directions were made.[31] In some cases, this created more problems for the employer than the original labour shortage. A personnel manager in an armaments factory recounted to MO the problems that arose from unskilled, inexperienced young women being sent to his factory, explaining that one new recruit 'came to my office in tears almost and near breaking-point. The noise, the smell of oil, coupled with the nervous and emotional strain of the past day or two had got her down. Spent another half-hour getting her calmed down, sent her home for the afternoon.'[32] In other cases, workers finding their job uncongenial might persistently turn up late or not at all. As a Welfare Manager explained, 'A worker can always get another job, but an employer has the devil of a job to replace a man especially if he is experienced in some special job.'[33] Such problems were a source of frustration and challenge to managers, and the war economy, but also to fellow workers who unsurprisingly became disgruntled at picking up the slack left by others. The same Welfare Manager commented on this knock-on effect: 'the awkward ones cause a disproportionate amount of trouble ... foremen have a misery of being unable to enforce discipline. They have to tolerate a worker who is idle or loses time for the sake of the bit of work that he or she does bother to do.'[34]

One reason for such disaffection was the nature of the work itself and the frequent mismatch between worker capability and actual tasks. One young woman who had been used to working in jobs that used her evident intelligence found herself in a Royal Ordnance factory and complained, 'It's the most footling silly work you can imagine. I consider I have a fair degree of intelligence and I am willing to use my capabilities for the war effort, but apparently the only thing they can use me for is to sit in an overheated room in front of a large machine and flick little nuts off a rod! If I thought about the job I'd just go haywire.'[35] A 1943 report by MO on factory work quoted another woman's complaint: 'I'd like to do it properly – learn to do a more complicated job. You don't feel you're doing nothing like this. Of course, we know it helps, but you know what I mean – you don't feel you're doing anything.'[36] Work that appeared meaningless and offered little in the way of satisfaction or purpose inevitably led women to be 'browned off'. Such an experience contrasts strongly with the ways in which a negative work environment could be part of a positive construction of masculinity, discussed in the last chapter. Here there was no sense that the attributes of the work, often meaningless and simplistic as they were, could in any way contribute to a constructive female working identity. That they fitted with an institutional and even governmental view that 'women's limited capabilities rendered them tolerant of boredom' highlights the limitations of the state's approach to work motivation and goes some way to explain many women's frustrations and the resulting psychological responses that could lead to absenteeism.[37]

However, it was not only women who sometimes struggled with the mismatch between ability and work, as an MO respondent wrote in her diary in 1943. She described the example of a friend's husband who had been a commercial artist before the war but ended up in a wartime factory doing manual labour and was 'thoroughly browned off, because once he started at this factory he has not been allowed to leave it'. She went on to explain that friends of his in similar positions had managed to swap their factory work for relevant draughtsmanship work in the Admiralty, but he was stuck in the factory and looked ten years older than when she'd last seen him. As well as the sense of frustration at the mismatch of capability and work and disappointment at the perceived lower status of his job, another key reason for his mental distress was the physical impact of the role, and particularly the long hours of work: 'At one time he was doing more than 60 hours a week, with three hours a day travelling, 1½ hrs – each end', she explained.[38] Such physically hard work, coupled with long and often disrupted commuting, undoubtedly took their toll on both the physical and mental health of many wartime workers, male and female. The tiredness and unhappiness that this created thus compounded any feelings of strain and exacerbated the stressful nature of people's day-to-day lives, and in turn had a detrimental effect on the economy through worker sickness and absenteeism.

Daily strain

Indeed, for many workers, regardless of gender, the simple struggle to get to work and back compounded the strain of long hours at work. As one Surrey aircraft worker explained, 'We have now been compelled to travel by train, which involves men and women being away from home 13 and 15 hours a day in order to do a mere 8½ hours. In my own case I am away from home 84 hours a week and can only do 55 hours, that is assuming the train is punctual in the morning, and very often it is not.'[39] A young woman told MO's researchers, 'At the bus stop it's like a mob, the men jump on the bus while it's going, and the women don't stand a chance. I can never get to work in time, I'm always late because I've waited so long for the bus.'[40] Such problems with transport created tension for the worker worrying about being late but were also a source of physical exhaustion as highlighted by the aircraft worker's account of his long days. *People in Production* summed up, 'Even before the war getting to and from work was one of the biggest friction points of the British industrial set-up', so additional wartime difficulties were 'making workers feel "browned off"'.[41]

For women, such transport problems aggravated another source of considerable wartime stress: 'The Shopping Problem', as MO's researchers called it.[42] Shopping was a challenge for most people during war, but for women workers performing a dual working role inside and outside the home, it was a very particular source of 'nervous strain'.[43] As one woman explained, 'We are expected to shop in the lunch hour, and that means either not having the proper lunch or not shopping properly.' For others, even this was impossible if they lived too far away from their place of work: 'it takes too long to get back and shop even if I spend the whole lunch hour on it'.[44] For many women their ration books were registered with shops near their homes, and often there were no relevant shops near to their places of work. Additionally, as another explained, 'It's all the extra things. You have to go to all the shops every day to see what they've got in, you've got to see that with a family to feed.'[45] Clearly this just was not possible for those working long hours, full-time, and as a result some women simply absented themselves from work in order to catch up with shopping or other household work. As one woman explained, 'I have to take a day off now and then … the work accumulates, that I must stay and put things right.'[46] Arguably such a break was an absolute necessity simply to shop, do housework and look after their own and, if they had them, their children's basic welfare. But even with a break, the combination of paid work and domestic responsibilities still led to fatigue and tension.[47] As MO had identified as early as 1940 in a report on 'Women and Morale', life on the Home Front for women was as onerous as military service was for men, albeit in different ways: 'The housewife, though she has not the direct leadership and discipline that the soldier experiences, may have to undergo more danger and put up with more inconveniences than her husband.'[48] Such inconveniences when compounded with the long hours (and often tedium) of work, unsurprisingly led to physical and mental strain, resulting in considerable absenteeism.

The authors of *People in Production*, while accepting the very real nature of such difficulties were, however, still critical of the workforce's apparent willingness to succumb to common afflictions as an excuse for absenteeism, stating, 'we can hardly fail to be impressed by what we can only call a massive latent hypochondria'. This they blamed on the pernicious effects of patent medicine advertising, arguing that 'a lot of illness wouldn't make people feel ill if they didn't have so much superficial knowledge now about the common afflictions'.[49] Such knowledge came from more than simply patent medicine advertising, however. Adverts in national newspapers for Cadbury's Bourn-vita hot drink emphasised its efficacy in promoting sleep and linked this to nervous conditions, labelling its ingredients as 'nerve-restoratives' and exhorting readers to 'Make up your mind that from now on you're going to have HEALTHY nerves – nerve-fitness is as important as physical fitness now.'[50] Similarly, testimonials for Yeast-Vite tablets in newspaper adverts included a bus conductor whose nerves 'gave way' and a woman who had 'been ill with nerves for a very long time'. Both highlighted additional physical ills and the small print of the advertisement suggested that the tablets were a remedy for 'Headaches, Neuralgia, Rheumatism, Nerves, Indigestion, Sleeplessness, Constipation.'[51] The MO researchers' view was that knowledge derived from these sorts of sources enabled workers to label and medically legitimise the feelings of discomfort, stress and worry resulting from wartime conditions. Arguably, what the language of advertising provided was culturally acceptable descriptions of a range of ailments that people could appropriate to explain, and more easily admit their physical and mental distress. Among the most frequently mentioned health complaints were coughs and colds, but workers also cited 'feelings of debility and tiredness' and 'increased nerviness' as well as 'stomach troubles, including ulcers and constipation'.[52] The latter physical explanations were often viewed as more 'respectable' justifications for both illness and visiting the doctor, particularly for men.[53] Dietary restrictions due to rationing as well as the simple strain of wartime life were also blamed for illness. The frequency of gastric problems and particularly ulcers in both the military and civilian populations during the war became a focus of much medical research and, as Miller has argued, helped popularise the idea that psychological states, such as wartime anxiety, were part of their cause, and thus psychotherapeutic as well as physiological treatments should be used.[54] This increased incidence of gastric problems during the war has also been seen as an example of the way in which a variety of cultural forces can come together to focus on a particular health issue, causing patients and doctors alike to give greater consideration to certain symptoms, and to foster widely shared beliefs about causes, resulting in an apparent increase in cases.[55]

However, according to MO's researchers, such worker complaints were preventable while the result of such hypochondria was clear: 'over thirty million weeks are lost each year in peacetime'.[56] The implication was that this was not something which could be tolerated by a nation at war. Yet the researchers were also aware of potential mitigating factors, explaining that 'the man or woman doing a real job of work needs (psychologically as much as physically) a relax right away from work, from time to time'. However, this was increasingly difficult to obtain, with 'holidays discouraged by the Government, and with normal holiday and recreational facilities severely cut by the war'. Thus workers simply took things into their own hands and responded with absenteeism so that 'Despite double-time on Sundays, many firms have had to give up working over weekends, or to make arrangements ensuring at least one day's break per week per worker.'[57] So while *People in Production*'s authors essentially dismissed both the mental distress of workers and the physical ailments that might result from that distress as a problem of the worker psyche, ailments which were effectively self-inflicted if not imagined, workers themselves took matters into their own hands to cope with the demands of wartime work.

Worker welfare

At the same time that MO was carrying out its research in factories around Britain, the *British Medical Journal* (*BMJ*) was also engaged with the topic of how to better manage worker health, reporting its concern that Britain's health services had 'not given enough consideration to the varying physical and psychological factors within factories and business organisations which can so profoundly affect health'.[58] The proposed solution, according to a further report in the same issue, included more emphasis on prevention and a closer association of the medical profession and industry.[59] However, despite the Factories (Medical and Welfare) Order of July 1940 requiring the appointment of doctors in factories involved with war production, the response to a parliamentary question of 1942 showed that only 'about a hundred whole-time and four hundred part-time doctors had been appointed to works since the Order'.[60] Furthermore, according to the *BMJ*, while such doctors had 'done much to improve health in industry', this had mainly been in larger firms that could afford them, and thus such benefits had 'often not been fully available for the great mass of workers'.[61]

It was not just the appointment of medical staff into organisations that was mooted as an answer to worker problems. There was also the provision of 'welfare', a fluid concept that tends to adapt and be adapted to the political and industrial climate of the day.[62] The wartime political and industrial climate in question undoubtedly framed it as whatever might improve worker morale, reduce absenteeism and increase production. As such, welfare took a myriad of forms. As the *People in Production* authors explained, 'Everything to do with human interests of workers in the factory, including the treatment of their injuries, the feeding of them, any entertainments that may be provided, pension schemes, sports clubs, comes under the heading of Welfare.'[63] However, they also suggested that welfare was something '*added on* to the factory in Britain, mostly added on recently and still to a minority'.[64] They warned, 'Welfare is a vague word in the industrial vocabulary with a somewhat pious, Salvation Army tang to it' with 'limiting and confusing associations.'[65] In practice, the worker's response to that sort of welfare often confounded the intention. As one Midlands factory worker explained with relief after leaving a workplace famous for its welfare, 'You couldn't call your soul your own, they *welfared you to death*.'[66] Female Welfare officers, especially those who were of a higher social class and emphasised discipline, were often perceived as 'nosy-parkers' and resentfully 'strung along'.[67] MO acknowledged that 'Welfare which is merely given out from above, is accepted in that spirit, and frequently distrusted for that reason.'[68]

The *People in Production* authors claimed that welfare existed in about half of the factories they reported on, adding, 'But in a great many of these it is thought of as something *purely physical*. In others it is a system of "patronage".'[69] In explaining this, it argued that many managements found it difficult to adopt even formal welfare and that even that was limited, recognising 'that the worker has an inside (a stomach for instance) as well as an outside. But often the recognition stops at the neck.' The account went on to highlight that both mind and body were critical to 'the something nowadays called morale – in normal times feeling, interest and attitude' and that it was this morale that was critical to the war effort.[70] An account from an Assistant Manager illustrated the problem. He explained that his firm had 'all the outward trappings of welfare', listing a canteen, cheap food, staff doctor and nurses, and pension and sickness visitor schemes. Staff were

> very well treated from the physical point of view and remuneration. Individually, they hardly exist. The management is benevolent but interested in technology and statistics rather than in individuals. What the staff want is human contact with the management, discussion about the future prospects of the individual and of the firm, a man-to-man outlook. What they get is notices pinned on the board.[71]

This was exacerbated by a general distrust of welfare initiatives by the unions, who suspected that workers were 'being "tricked"' and that welfare was a 'device by management to please workers and yet keep down their economic standard'.[72] Such suspicion of employers' welfare provisions was not new: J. B. Priestley had drawn attention to Cadbury's extensive welfare in his *English Journey* of 1934, criticising its 'falsely mystical aura' and arguing for 'workers combining to provide these benefits, or a reasonable proportion of them, for themselves ... far removed from the factory'.[73] Implied was a concern that any welfare provision and apparent care for the well-being of the worker merely represented the forces of capital protecting their profit by mollifying potential worker disruption through an excess of benevolence. Similarly, attempts by psychologists and health workers to engage the Trade Union Congress (TUC) in research on psychoneuroses in the 1930s were largely ignored, perhaps because the TUC was reluctant to acknowledge that their members' health problems might result from psychological causes.[74]

A Welfare Officer's casebook

Despite such misgivings, many organisations went to some lengths to comply with welfare legislation, including the appointment of designated Welfare Officers, such as Miss Richmond. She was the Welfare Officer for Hunter and Sons, a London furnishings business with premises and small business concerns all over London, including four factories in Houndsditch, Victoria, Acton and Battersea during the war.[75] The following section examines her reports of visits to sick employee, some of them suffering from work-related nervous conditions, between 1943 and 1956. While her job was to give assistance and support to employees who were on sick leave, her reports on her visits also illustrate the role that colleagues and family played in enabling or preventing the individual from acknowledging or understanding their stress. They also highlight considerable continuity in framing stress as a problem of the individual worker.

Miss Richmond's job involved her in a range of activities, including visiting absent workers at home and in hospital, and she displayed compassion and concern for many of the people she supported. However, her response to some of the nervous cases suggests a limit to her compassion and a view of mental health that was both gendered and firmly situated within the individualised concept of responsibility dominant at the time. Her stance included sympathy for the nervous but also a level of scepticism about conditions that were so difficult to understand for the non-sufferer and that for many were also associated with feelings of fear and shame. In 1949 she wrote up her report of her visit to a Mr Adams who was 'suffering from what is called, I suppose, a nervous breakdown', and detailed what she had told him:

> Business worries are a dreadful nervous ordeal whilst they are happening: they seem to accumulate and no end can be seen. But once the end has come – bad or good isn't the point, the fact that it has ended is what matters – the time for a nervous breakdown is over. One must just get on with things, life goes on, that worry is over. There may be others in the future, who knows? Deal with them when they come but don't dwell on what is past.[76]

Her words imply a certain impatience with Mr Adams's continuing struggle with his nerves. Earlier in the report she had outlined the cause of his problems, explaining that he had taken over the work of a surveyor who had left the organisation and discovered that three existing orders were muddled and creating a financial loss for Hunters: 'This worried Mr Adams considerably and as the financial losses increased with the progress of the work so did his worry, until it overwhelmed him and he had a nervous breakdown.' Despite reassurance from his managers, 'the worry had taken too great a hold' of Mr Adams and he was now 'suffering from his nerves'.[77]

Despite usually showing considerable compassion for the many workers she visited, Miss Richmond revealed an attitude that had much in common with the authors of *People in Production*'s comments on hypochondria, after visiting Mr Adams and another employee, Mr Croft, who was also suffering from nerves. Her reported started, 'What a week and what an object lesson!!!!!! To listen to these two grown men telling me how their "nerves" have gone to pieces because the "worry of their work has got on top of them" and so on and on and on and on.'[78] Her pointed reference to 'grown men' is a telling illustration of gendered understandings of mental distress and seems also to suggest that she saw their inability to manage their worrying as somehow childish. Such notions are consistent with the idea that it was the sufferer's weakness rather than external conditions that were at the heart of their condition. While MO's *People in Production* considered much worker illness as hypochondria, it did include some acknowledgement of the contribution of external factors such as shopping and transport problems to workers 'nerves'.[79] Miss Richmond continued her report by setting out her views quite robustly, perhaps revealing her own level of frustration and strain in dealing with such cases:

> Many illnesses, pneumonia etc cannot be helped and nobody falls and breaks a leg on purpose, but I have seen so much of this 'nervous breakdown' line and it is a thing that the individual can prevent – if taken in time. The red light is showing when you find yourself thinking about, and talking about, nothing else than your particular worry. Mental diversion is needed: people, amusements, hobbies, anything except sitting brooding and chain smoking. Above all get away. Weekends, even only Sundays, get away. The problem doesn't go but the mind is steadied and the person is able to regain a sense of proportion and see the problem for what it is; certainly something quite normal and capable of being dealt with. To hear these 'nerve' people talk one would think it was a question of life or death confronting them. They are quite out of focus with reality. It is no use talking to cases like these two I have seen this week. They are too far gone.[80]

Notable are her comments on prevention which reflected a common view of personal responsibility, also seen in the self-help books examined in the first chapter. Essentially, she saw the sufferer as complicit in their own suffering due to weakness or self-indulgence in worry. In another case, she reported her conversation with the sister of Mr Brown, a storekeeper at the subsidiary firm Shaws, who had 'been in hospital for the last three weeks receiving treatment for "nervous trouble"'. He had suffered the same 'illness' two years earlier when he was a costing clerk and, on that occasion, had been hospitalised for several months. According to Miss Richmond, Mr Brown's sister claimed, 'she did not think it had been right because he was working under the man who had his old job and he had had an inferiority complex all the time: he is now "just a bundle of nerves, there is nothing wrong with him physically, it is something to do with his work that has got him like this"'.[81] Mr Brown's sister's insistence that his condition was *not* physical, but related to his work was unusual among contemporary accounts, but perhaps attributable to an attempt to ensure the firm took responsibility and kept him on.

Miss Richmond concluded her report with robust pragmatism: 'It is a sad case and I am sorry for the Browns but, after all, Shaws is not a Psychiatric Rehabilitation Centre for the employment of "nervous trouble" cases. They did try to help Mr Brown but are now back where they were two years ago when he had a similar "nervous breakdown". Who can tell when another "breakdown" will occur?'[82]

Miss Richmond's own role and her considerable itinerary of hospital visits, and what amounted to informal social work amongst the employees, seem to suggest a level of compassion and care by her employer. Yet even the most paternalistic employer had limits, both in terms of keeping jobs open during sick leave and in admitting any culpability. The fact that Mr Brown had been returned to a demoted role in the same area he had worked in before shows a disregard for any contributing factor his working environment might have had on his condition. This disconnect between the experience of the worker and the effect of the work or workplace was simply a case of ignoring a problem which both employer and worker wished to downplay: workers because they relied on their job for survival, and for many the spectre of the Depression still loomed large, and employers because it did not register as their responsibility. If you were ill that was your problem and in such circumstances it seems fair to conjecture that many whose work caused stress were scarcely able to acknowledge it themselves. Indeed, the organisation's apparent caring paternalism may be interpreted more coldly as self-interest, as labour shortages during and after the war meant employers were keen to hang on to experienced employees, even if that meant enduring a period of sick leave. Certainly, the scale of Miss Richmond's visiting, for example, 412 visits on 179 days in 1945, and the length of some employee absences could support either interpretation.[83] Despite this, in many ways, Miss Richmond's work at Hunters represented the positive end of the scale in terms of employer responses to worker stress. And while the organisation might still frame that stress as inherent to the worker rather than their work or working environment, it was at least being acknowledged and addressed.

Roffey Park Rehabilitation Centre

As an example of the kind of organisational welfare that really did look at workers as individuals, the experiment at Roffey Park in West

Sussex proved a serious, but short-lived attempt to deal with stressed workers during the war. The Centre was a private concern created specifically to deal with cases of industrial neurosis (here used as a catch-all label incorporating any nervous condition relating to a work context) with the explicit aim of getting workers back to health and back to work. It offered treatment for workers and training and education for Personnel Managers and other relevant professionals, while also pursuing a similar agenda to the MRC research of the 1930s by trying to categorise and establish criteria for identifying employees who were potentially vulnerable to industrial neurosis. Created towards the end of the war, its attempts at a scalable approach to work stress were ultimately hampered by cost and the variable nature, complexity and divergent causes of workplace stress. Analysis of the work at Roffey Park suggests that such attempts continued to grapple with the issue of what actually constituted industrial neurosis or work-related nerves, with the Centre's own report describing the conditions it was targeting as 'industrial fatigue, depression, anxiety states and other manifestations of indeterminate ill-health', the last noticeably incorporating a huge range of potential ills.[84] The Centre's work also revealed that some workplace stress had little to do with work at all and its efforts to identify categories of susceptible workers were more revealing of the social and cultural prejudices of researchers than of conclusive and useful classifications.

The Centre at Roffey Park was established in 1943 by the NCRIW with the support of St Thomas' Hospital in London. The NCRIW was made up of representatives from medicine and industry chaired by Lord Horder, personal physician to the king, and president of the Peckham Health Centre, with Samuel Courtauld of the textile company and founder of the Courtauld Institute of Art as vice chairman. Acute labour shortages and concerns about lost industrial production through 'breakdowns in health or efficiency' prompted the decision of the NCRIW to buy two adjoining estates in West Sussex and create a centre for rehabilitating workers. Promoted by Horder and Courtauld, the centre was funded by members of the NCRIW, including Courtaulds, Cable & Wireless, the Co-operative Wholesale Society, Vauxhall Motors and Ericsson Telephones to name but a few.[85] Financial contributions varied from a considerable £5,000 (from Courtaulds) to £3 3s from Energen Foods Ltd. The Centre's stated aim was to provide residential treatment for 'the multiple cases of indeterminate ill-health arising from industrial fatigue, depression, nervous debility and other occupational or psychological disorders, with the object of returning as many workers as possible to a full-time productive capacity'.[86] Its ethos centred around modern treatments and research within a democratic atmosphere, including the housing of all resident members of staff in one accommodation building, rather than separate facilities for doctors, nurses and administrative staff.[87]

Its target patient population was wide and unsurprisingly priority for admission was given to employees of subscribing organisations. According to *The Lancet*, reporting on the Centre in 1945, its patients were drawn from 'managers, secretaries and accountants, as well as from those who earn their living with their hands; and this mixing of people from a wide range of economic and social backgrounds has never presented any difficulties; it has, in fact, benefited both patient and community'.[88] Patients might come to Roffey Park for a number of reasons, as *The Lancet* explained:

> The quiet sensible man, after twenty years of steady service, may become depressed, bewildered, unable to concentrate or to complete his ordinary day's work; the young man or woman beginning to take responsibility may be overwhelmed by domestic or emotional disasters; the energetic, methodical middle-aged secretary may develop obsessional fears; and for others life is spoiled by morbid anxiety.[89]

It is notable that in its own descriptions, the Centre made little reference to the direct impact of war on occupational stresses and strains, although later descriptions of some inmates refer to their particular wartime experiences. This may have been a deliberate omission intended to frame the Centre's work in a way which would enable its continuation after the war. Recognising that the people who were referred there were 'often a serious problem' not just for industrial doctors, but other organisational professionals too, such as 'works managers, personnel managers, trade union officials and social workers from hospitals', Roffey Park very quickly became a centre for their education, its Training Department opening in 1947 and several five- and two-day residential courses held in the first year for 354 people.[90]

Despite enthusiasm for both treating industrial nervous conditions and educating employers and doctors, there was recognition that defining what was being treated was problematic. As the Centre's advisory panel reported in 1949, 'The type of case admitted has been referred to as "industrial" neurosis, but this is a loose expression which has no medical significance and can mean nothing beyond the fact that the patient has been engaged in some form of work.'[91] Notwithstanding this apparent vagueness, there was a full programme of treatment. As the *BMJ* reported in an article co-authored by Roffey Park's Medical Director, Dr Thomas Ling in 1950, '"Talking out" of problems, "counselling" techniques, and narco-analysis are extensively employed. Electric convulsion therapy, modified insulin therapy, and other physical methods of treatment are utilised where necessary.'[92] The emphasis on talking therapies contrasts with their apparent absence in contemporary self-help books noted in Chapter 1 and with the cultural norm of reticence regarding mental health issues. Perhaps even more significant was the use of potentially dangerous physical treatments, particularly when the advisory panel report seemed to suggest a certain level of imprecision about diagnosis.[93] The Centre's own booklet published in 1946 emphasised that 'each case is fully investigated by one of the three resident doctors and suitable medical, psychological and occupational treatment is arranged. Visiting specialists are available if required.'[94] Such emphasis on thoroughness was a vital reassurance in the face of the potentially dangerous physical treatments, as well as a necessity in dealing with a condition that could vary so much between patients.

Photographs in one of Roffey Park's publicity booklets showed patients at work on machines in a workshop, and were captioned, 'The other fellow's job provides interest and relaxation to workers from a different sphere'; others showed them taking part in physical exercise, gardening or after-dinner discussions, placing the emphasis more on occupational therapy than medical intervention.[95] The described regime proposed a rather utopian vision of communal living:

> All patients take part in the work of the Centre, they are responsible for keeping their own rooms tidy, assisting in the kitchen and dining hall while occupational workshops and gardens give a complete change from normal routine and surroundings. Meals are planned by a trained dietitian, including fresh fruit and vegetables from the ten acres under cultivation ... the patients are encouraged to help in the cultivation of produce under the instruction of a Horticulturist.[96]

Evening leisure time was catered for by 'educational films, discussion groups, brains trusts, concerts, dances and talks of general interest by qualified speakers'.[97] It seems likely that after years of wartime hardships either in military service or on the Home Front, the opportunity of six weeks at Roffey Park away from responsibilities, eating a superior diet and enjoying interesting pastimes, was likely to benefit *anyone's* well-being, mental and physical. However, in a discussion about industrial doctors' approaches to worker breakdowns, *The Lancet* acknowledged that while time and opportunity would enable recovery, for most 'it may not be easy for the firm to spare them for long without replacing them'.[98]

Organisations might be reluctant to allow an employee opportunity to recover, but in some cases, it was their own fault that a problem had arisen. The case of May B, described in Roffey Park's course booklet, described a typist suffering from depression and insomnia attributed to overwork, and showed that it was her employer's failure to address a known personnel problem that led to her stay at the Centre: 'there had been serious difficulties in her department for some months. The woman in charge was irrational, difficult and liable to have favourites, with the result that there had been marked difficulties in obtaining the required additional staff. A vicious circle had thus been produced which was the important factor in May's ill-health.' Once this was addressed, the case study went on to confirm that 'after a few weeks May went back to work. Six months later she was reported to be well and working happily.'[99] In other cases, it transpired that illness had little to do with an individual's work and everything to do with the difficulties of readjusting to civilian life after being a prisoner of war. Thus, Robert W was 'admitted complaining of inability to settle into work. Before the war, he had been employed satisfactorily as a clerk in the City and during the war saw action in North Africa and Italy.' The case study went on to explain that he was a prisoner of war for two years in Germany and since returning had had five unsatisfactory jobs and 'On admission he was tense, irritable, hypercritical and sleeping badly. Physically his nutrition was poor and some of his teeth septic.' Once treatment was begun this 'showed that much of his trouble was due to half-forgotten experiences as a prisoner of war'. Tests revealed that Robert W had good mechanical aptitude, so while being treated he was 'placed in the wood workshop, where he made good progress.

After some weeks he had lost his irritability, was mixing well with the other patients and was sleeping without drugs.'[100] Arrangements were made for him to be trained as a carpenter by the Ministry of Labour and enquiry twelve months later showed that he was employed satisfactorily on house construction.[101]

The crucial point is that Robert W and others were treated for symptoms supposedly arising due to work because it was only within the context of work that their symptoms had meaning and cultural validity. Undoubtedly, plenty of other ex-servicemen struggled to readjust to civilian life, but if their symptoms arose in social or domestic settings rather than at work, they were more likely to be ignored or denied. For some, it was likely to be less problematic to relate psychological problems to work than to having served one's country in war. Certainly, the military and governments preferred it that way when it came to paying out pensions to psychological casualties.[102] Similarly, domestic strains that could not be expressed *in situ* might appear at work, as the case of Margaret S, a dispenser in a chemist shop, showed: 'On admission she was found to be in poor general health and very introspective. Further enquiry revealed an unsatisfactory situation both at home and at work, to which she was reacting adversely. Her home life was controlled by a dominating mother who treated her as a small child, with the result that she had no social outlets except at work.' Margaret responded well to treatment and 'arrangements were made for her to assist in the Research Laboratories of the Company, where she could live in a hostel and work under good, hygienic conditions. The mother was seen also, and her cooperation secured so that the girl could lead a fuller social life.'[103] Like Robert W, the manifestation of her problems at work gave them a validity which enabled treatment. However, amongst the great mass of the British workforce, these few cases were exceptional in having been identified and referred to Roffey Park.

Used in Roffey Park's own publicity materials, these case studies highlight the focus of both the Centre and its subscribing organisations: the recovery of the worker. To some extent, the nature of their condition was immaterial and thus it did not matter that industrial neurosis was a 'loose expression' as the Centre simply treated whatever psychological (and physical) problems were presented. While understandable when organisational focus was on wartime productivity, this was not ultimately a sustainable organisational solution. At the very least it was expensive, costing £4 14s 6d per week (roughly equivalent to a week's wages) for maintenance, with an average stay lasting six weeks.[104] According to the *BMJ* 33.8 per cent of the 512 patients treated in 1948 and who responded to a follow-up letter indicated they were much improved, with 44.7 per cent improved and 21.5 per cent unimproved. Follow-up responses from industrial medical officers on eighty-five cases were even more positive with 54.1 per cent much improved and working full-time, 37.7 per cent improved and working full-time, and only 8.2 per cent unimproved or had left the company. Of the cases followed up, 28 per cent did not elicit a reply, and the authors suggested 'some of these ex-patients are unlikely to be well, but some who are now well wish to forget their nervous illness and will not answer as they wish to sever contact with the hospital'.[105] Despite the pragmatic approach to industrial neurosis and the apparent success of the treatment, even Roffey Park doctors had to admit that any mental illness still carried a considerable stigma. To that end, its training programme offered advice and guidance for those working with and managing nervous workers, aimed at equipping them to deal with the problems encountered by rehabilitated employees.

Professional training

Research and training were understood to be a key part of the Centre's role, aimed at disseminating ideas to both industry and health services: a role that became even more important after the war ended and it became clear that treatment would be integrated into the NHS.[106] Training for industrial medical staff, personnel and union officials at Roffey Park focused on two elements: '1. the maintenance of fitness at work and 2. special problems of rehabilitation and resettlement.'[107] The latter focused particularly on categories of patients believed to have their own specific requirements, including ex-servicemen, the disabled, gastric and neurosis cases, and one or two other 'special examples' such as 'the chronic "grouser"' and 'the social misfit'.[108] These categories were also reflected in publications by the doctors working at Roffey Park, including Dr Roger Tredgold, Boots Lecturer in Industrial Health. His book *Human Relations in Modern Industry* contained a chapter on specific susceptible workers, including, in its 1949 edition, the 'dullard', 'the accident-prone', the 'returned wanderer', the 'refugee' and eventually, in its 1963 version, the 'ageing worker and executive'.[109] Such categorisations appear simplistic and pejorative in retrospect and failed to acknowledge issues of motivation, despite Tredgold's own stated view that this was determined by more than just money. Instead he argued that certain kinds of work ('drudgery') should be done by 'dullards perhaps – or perhaps those whose parents have given them less education'.[110] Nor was he really offering any tangible methods of dealing with the identified categories, beyond drawing the attention of personnel and welfare managers (his intended readership) to their existence.

What his work does suggest strongly is that both the medical profession and employers approached the propensity to work-related stress as being inherent to the individual. Where they did recognise environmental factors, such as the poor supervisor in May B's case, the emphasis was still on the individual's predisposition. This implies an ongoing reluctance to consider their accountability for the worker's organisational environment and a continuing emphasis on personal rather than organisational responsibility, whatever good intentions might be driving such research. It was far easier to assume that the problem lay with the individual due to some innate weakness than in what was being asked of them as a worker. That is not to say that the training offered at Roffey Park and publications such as Tredgold's were not helpful in educating a range of key people in organisations, including trade unionists, of the potential for work stress, but such education remained largely in the hands of those whose main task was to mitigate, remove or avoid hiring such workers. They might be alert to the signs of stress in workers, but ironically workers themselves did not necessarily have the information or knowledge to recognise signs in themselves or to realise that such signs might be acknowledgeable.

The pressing necessity of maintaining worker health to ensure production during the war and immediate post-war period was undoubtedly the driver for the creation of Roffey Park, although the welfarism that Priestley criticised before the war was also a contributory factor.[111] There is little doubt that the workers who were sent to Roffey Park benefited, but it was certainly not altruism which drove their employers to provide such a service. Nevertheless, one specialist centre was undoubtedly limited in its effect, and although the interested parties envisaged an industrial and occupational health service forming part of the nascent

NHS, this did not come to fruition, largely because of the division of health responsibilities between ministries when the NHS was established.[112] More obviously, the imprecision of industrial neurosis as a diagnosis and the length and expense of treatment must have made arguing for specific work-related psychiatric centres unrealistic against a backdrop of limited general psychiatric provision. As the Treasurer of the NCRIW himself noted in a confidential letter about Roffey Park and psychiatry in general to a member of the St Thomas' Hospital Board, 'neurosis beds are in short supply'.[113] This ultimately doomed Roffey Park's long-term specialist status and it was swiftly subsumed into the NHS as a general psychiatric hospital until its closure in 1983.[114]

Conclusion

In the build-up to the Second World War, the authorities in Britain had anticipated and planned for extensive psychiatric casualties resulting from aerial warfare. When such casualties did not materialise, this was largely taken to show that the British public was more psychologically resilient than had been assumed. Where there was acknowledgement of the potential psychological effect of wartime conditions, in propaganda such as the leaflet 'Just Nerves!' it involved a somewhat contradictory message advising people to seek help, while also reminding them that many people felt the same and that they should not use any nervous suffering as an excuse to shirk their duties. Such wartime stress was therefore framed as a normal response to conditions, but one that must simply be endured and overcome by the individual. Underlying this was a sense that one could acknowledge the effects of war on one's psyche, but only *in extremis* could any sort of treatment or respite be justified. Research by MO into wartime factory production and particularly problems of absenteeism and motivation effectively revealed that while many people did adopt a stoic approach to life on the Home Front, the mundane and everyday challenges of that existence created an underlying strain that either led to physical illness or was explained via the proxy of physical complaints and fuelled the absenteeism that so troubled organisations and government alike. The provision of 'welfare' in various forms was intended to address this. Miss Richmond's work as a Welfare Officer in a London concern illustrates both how the role functioned, but also popularly held beliefs about those suffering from work-related nervous conditions that framed their suffering as essentially self-inflicted. Similarly, the research carried out during the brief existence of the Rehabilitation Centre at Roffey Park and in its more long-lived training facility also tended to focus on the innate qualities of the worker, particularly in trying to identify and categorise susceptible workers. At the same time, patient examples from the Centre suggested that while a diagnosis of industrial neurosis might arise within a work context, causes could originate elsewhere. In such cases, the context of work gave validity to suffering that might otherwise either have been ignored, or that was perhaps too problematic to acknowledge within a domestic setting. Yet for many, particularly women, the domestic environment and the double-duty role of work inside and outside the home was increasingly being recognised as a cause of stress.

Notes

1 Tom Harrisson, *Living through the Blitz* (London: Collins, 1976), p. 102. Italics in the original.
2 Corinna Peniston-Bird and Penny Summerfield. '"Hey, You're Dead!". The Multiple Use of Humour in Representations of British National Defence in the Second World War', *Journal of European Studies* 31, 123 (2001); p. 413, https://doi.org/10.1177/004724410103112314.
3 Shephard, *War of Nerves*, p. 174.
4 Richard Morris Titmuss, *Problems of Social Policy* (London: H.M.S.O., 1950), p. 20.
5 Robert Mackay, *Half the Battle: Civilian Morale in Britain during the Second World War* (Manchester; New York: Manchester University Press, 2002), pp. 80, 174. Humphrey Jennings and Harry Watt, *Britain Can Take It* (GPO Film Unit, 1940). *Britain Can Take It* was a Ministry of Information-sponsored film showing the resilience of Londoners during one night of the Blitz.
6 FR 926, Summary of Talk to the British Psychological Society, 26 October 1941, MOA, University of Sussex, p. 1.
7 *Ibid.*, p. 7.
8 FR 739, Preliminary Report: Questionnaire on psychological war work and on air-raids, 4 May 1941, MOA, University of Sussex, p. 1.
9 Richard Overy, *The Bombing War: Europe 1939–1945* (London: Allen Lane, 2013), p. 169.
10 *Ibid.*, p. 170.
11 *Ibid.*, p. 171.

12 Harrisson, *Blitz*, p. 174.
13 Shephard, *War of Nerves*, p. 179.
14 For discussion of wartime morale and post-war construction of a mythologised wartime spirit, see Angus Calder, *The Myth of the Blitz* (London: Pimlico, 1992); Mackay, *Half the Battle*; Susan R. Grayzel, *At Home and Under Fire: Air Raids and Culture in Britain from the Great War to the Blitz* (Cambridge; New York: Cambridge University Press, 2011); Lucy Noakes and Juliette Pattinson (eds) *British Cultural Memory and the Second World War* (London: Bloomsbury, 2014).
15 Overy, *Bombing War*, p. 177.
16 Lucy Noakes, 'Gender, Grief, and Bereavement in Second World War Britain', *Journal of War & Culture Studies* 8, 1 (1 February 2015): p. 73, https://doi.org/10.1179/1752628014Y.0000000016.
17 Central Council, 'Just Nerves!'
18 FR 1629, Health Questionnaire, 24 March 1943, MOA, University of Sussex, pp. 2–3, 11.
19 FR 428, Report of Press Advertisements and Air Raids, 29 September 1940, MOA, University of Sussex, p. 1.
20 For example: 'You'll Stop Nagging Once You've Bought a Tin of "Peace-Time Sleep" Cadbury's Bourn-Vita Still at Peace-Time Prices', *Daily Mirror* (19 February 1940), p. 16; 'Collecting Fares in the Blackout Had Its Effect on Me: Trolley Bus Conductor Is Now "as Fit as Ever" Thanks to Yeast-Vite', *Daily Mirror* (27 August 1940), p. 6; 'When You Are "All Nerves": The Result of Worry and Anxiety Dr Williams Pink Pills', *Daily Mirror* (29 November 1940), p. 10.
21 Max Blyth, 'A History of the Central Council for Health Education 1927–1968' (PhD thesis, University of Oxford, 1987), p. 180.
22 Central Council, 'Just Nerves!'; Blyth, 'History of the CCHE', pp. 205–6, 209.
23 Central Council, 'Just Nerves!'
24 Angus Calder, *The People's War: Britain 1939–45* (London: Pimlico, 1992), pp. 538–9.
25 Central Council, 'Just Nerves!'
26 Sonya O. Rose, *Which People's War? National Identity and Citizenship in Wartime Britain 1939–1945* (Oxford: Oxford University Press, 2003), p. 185.
27 *Ibid.*, p. 109.
28 *An Enquiry into British War Production – A Report Prepared by Mass Observation for the Advertising Service Guild. Part 1: People in Production* (London: John Murray, 1942), p. viii.
29 *Ibid.*, pp. 6–9.

30 *Ibid.*, p. 256.
31 Calder, *People's War*, p. 235.
32 *People in Production*, p. 165.
33 *Ibid.*, p. 104.
34 *Ibid.*
35 *People in Production*, p. 156.
36 Tom Harrisson, *War Factory: A Report by Mass Observation* (London: Gollancz, 1943), p. 48.
37 Summerfield, *Women Workers*, p. 167.
38 D5311, 'Diary for 4 September' (1943), MOA, University of Sussex.
39 *People in Production*, p. 283.
40 *Ibid.*, p. 284.
41 *Ibid.*, pp. 280–4. Some forty years later the vagaries of British Rail remained stressful. As one bank worker told MO in 1983, 'I became unemployed as a result of a nervous breakdown in January directly attributable to the pressures of office work and travel by British Rail.' 'Replies to Summer directive Work' (1983), MOA, University of Sussex, H275.
42 *People in Production*, p. 226.
43 FR 520, Women and Morale, 10 December 1940, 7, MOA, University of Sussex, p. 7.
44 *People in Production*, p. 227.
45 *Ibid.*, p. 227.
46 *Ibid.*, p. 241.
47 Summerfield, *Women Workers*, pp. 135, 123.
48 MOA FR 520, Women and Morale, p. 2.
49 *People in Production*, p. 253.
50 'Peace-Time Sleep', *Daily Mirror*, p. 16.
51 'Collecting Fares in the Blackout', *Daily Mirror*, p. 6.
52 *People in Production*, p. 254.
53 Haggett, *Male Psychological Disorders*, p. 31.
54 Ian Miller, 'The Mind and Stomach at War: Stress and Abdominal Illness in Britain c.1939–1945', *Medical History* 54, 1 (2010): p. 108.
55 *Ibid.*, pp. 109–10.
56 *People in Production*, p. 257.
57 *Ibid.*, pp. 219–20.
58 Donald Stewart, 'Industrial Medical Services in Great Britain: A Critical Survey', *BMJ* II, 4221 (1941): p. 762, https://doi.org/10.1136/bmj.2.4221.762.
59 BMA Special Committee, 'Medical Supervision of Industrial Workers', *BMJ* II, 4221 (1941): p. 783, https://doi.org/10.1136/bmj.2.4221.783.

60 Stewart, 'Medical Services', p. 762.

61 *Ibid.*, p. 763.

62 Helen Jones, 'Employers' Welfare Schemes and Industrial Relations in Inter-War Britain', *Business History* 25, 1 (1983): p. 61, https://doi.org/10.1080/00076798300000005.

63 *People in Production*, p. 352.

64 *Ibid.*, pp. 352–3. Italics in the original.

65 *Ibid.*, p. 352.

66 *Ibid.*, p. 353. Italics in the original.

67 Summerfield, *Women Workers*, p. 128.

68 *People in Production*, p. 354.

69 *Ibid.*, p. 353. Italics in the original.

70 *Ibid.*, p. 354.

71 *Ibid.*, p. 353.

72 *Ibid.*, p. 359.

73 J. B. Priestley, *English Journey* (London: William Heinemann Ltd in association with Victor Gollancz Ltd, 1934), pp. 98, 100.

74 Vicky Long, *The Rise and Fall of the Healthy Factory: The Politics of Industrial Health in Britain, 1914–60* (Basingstoke: Palgrave Macmillan, 2011), p. 111.

75 'Papers of Miss Richmond' (1943 to 1956), Personal Collections, MOA, University of Sussex. With the exception of Miss Richmond, the names of all individuals and organisations have been replaced with pseudonyms at the request of the archivist.

76 'Welfare Visitor's Report', 22 September 1949, Papers of Miss Richmond, Personal Collections, MOA, University of Sussex.

77 'Welfare Visitor's Report 22/9/1949'.

78 *Ibid.*

79 *People in Production*, p. 227.

80 'Welfare Visitor's Report 22/9/1949'.

81 'Welfare Visitor's Report', 24 May 1954, Papers of Miss Richmond, Personal Collections, MOA, University of Sussex.

82 *Ibid.*

83 'Annual Report of Visits Made by Welfare Visitor (1945)' (January 1946), Papers of Miss Richmond, Personal Collections, MOA, University of Sussex.

84 National Council for the Rehabilitation of Industrial Workers, 'Roffey Park Rehabilitation Centre: A Record of Two Years' Progress, 1944–1946' (1946), Wellcome Library.

85 *Ibid.*

86 Roffey Park Institute Ltd, 'Health and Human Relations in Industry: The Courses at Roffey Park' (1947), Wellcome Library.

87 'A Rest From Industry', *The Lancet* 246, 6376 (10 November 1945): p. 608, https://doi.org/10.1016/S0140-6736(45)91627-8.

88 *Ibid.*, p. 607.

89 *Ibid.*

90 *Ibid.* Roffey Park Institute Ltd, 'Courses at Roffey Park'.

91 Roffey Park Rehabilitation Centre Advisory Panel, 'Confidential Report of the Advisory Panel Appointed by the Governors of St Thomas' Hospital in Connection with Roffey Park Rehabilitation Centre' (London: St Thomas' Hospital, 1949), Wellcome Library.

92 Thomas M. Ling, J. A. Purser and E. W. Rees, 'Incidence and Treatment of Neurosis in Industry', *BMJ* 2, 4671 (1950): p. 160, https://doi.org/jstor.org/stable/25357681.

93 Roffey Park Rehabilitation Centre Advisory Panel, 'Confidential Report'.

94 National Council for the Rehabilitation of Industrial Workers, 'Record of Two Years' Progress', p. 6.

95 *Ibid.*

96 NCRIW, 'Record of Two Years' Progress', p. 8.

97 *Ibid.*

98 'A Rest From Industry', p. 607.

99 Roffey Park Institute Ltd, 'Courses at Roffey Park'.

100 *Ibid.*

101 *Ibid.*

102 Alan Allport, *Demobbed: Coming Home after the Second World War* (New Haven; London: Yale University Press, 2009), p. 196. Allport suggests that the War Office was keen to define psychological casualties as victims of pre-existing constitutional weakness rather than of military service in order to deny thousands of war pension claims.

103 Roffey Park Institute Ltd, 'Courses at Roffey Park'.

104 NCRIW, 'Record of Two Years' Progress'. £5 per week was a 'respectable working-class income' in Jim Tomlinson, 'Reconstructing Britain: Labour in Power 1945–1951', in Nick Tiratsoo (ed.) *From Blitz to Blair: A New History of Britain since 1939* (London: Weidenfeld & Nicolson, 1997), p. 95.

105 Ling, Purser and Rees, 'Incidence and Treatment of Neurosis in Industry', p. 161.

106 Roffey Park Institute Ltd, 'Courses at Roffey Park'.

107 *Ibid.*

108 *Ibid.*

109 Roger F. Tredgold, *Human Relations in Modern Industry* (London: Duckworth, 1949), p. 159. Roger F. Tredgold, *Human Relations in Modern Industry*, second and revised ed. (London: Gerald Duckworth & Co. Ltd, 1963), p. 127.

110 Tredgold, *Human Relations* (1949), p. 41.

111 Priestley, *English Journey*, pp. 98, 100.

112 Paul Weindling, 'Linking Self Help and Medical Science: The Social History of Occupational Health', in Paul Weindling (ed.) *The Social History of Occupational Health* (London; Sydney: Croom Helm, 1985), p. 16.

113 C. Harold Vernon, 'Confidential Letter to Hon. Arthur Howard', 1948, Roffey Park Rehabilitation Centre correspondence, memoranda and minutes of meetings 1948–1949, Wellcome Library.

114 W. John Giles, *The First Forty: Roffey Park Institute 1946–1987* (Roffey Park Institute, 1988), p. 30.

4

The great strain: domestic troubles in post-war Britain

In March 1942 MO received a letter from Mrs C, one of their volunteer respondents and diary keepers. She wrote to explain the gap in her contributions, blaming 'a bad mental breakdown against which I have been struggling for months! If you've read my diary, you must have noticed the great strain against which I've been working for months and months.'[1] A year later, after yet another gap in her submissions, she again sent an explanatory letter, this time citing a job change, but adding, 'Also, I was too, too utterly fed up to write. And then, as you know, I daren't write at home for fear my husband turned up and so I gave it up as a bad job.'[2] Mrs C worked as a nurse in Leeds, was married to Reg, and had two daughters. Between 1941 and 1944 she kept a sporadic diary for MO in which she detailed the strains of her unhappy marriage, as well as her daily existence as a housewife and her work as a nurse, first at the local hospital and then in a factory. Her letter of 1943 was indicative of her writings which, while chatty in tone, often dealt with the day-to-day stress of a difficult personal life: 'Life at home is more unbearable than ever. My husband will not be persuaded to believe me when I tell him that he does not mean a thing to me, and so we go on, dragging out this farce of a marriage.'[3] Her diaries bring to the fore her struggles to manage family resources, the demands of shift work, and Reg's often unannounced appearances on leave, all exacerbated by wartime shortages, their poor relationship and her involvement in an extra-marital love affair.

Domestic stress at the mid-century, as Mrs C's writings show, was largely expressed through references to strain, being fed up, nerves and even mental breakdown. As the examination of familial and household experiences and their cultural representations in the post-war period will show, while the term stress was still not used, the concept of a form of domestic stress was becoming increasingly visible in both popular and social scientific discourses. Although tensions within the home were by no means a new phenomenon, the increasing acknowledgement of such difficulties in public, their representation in popular culture and the growing professional interest in examining them, all contributed to the growth of the public stress discourse. A range of terminology that included nerves and breakdowns but also extended to notions of tiredness was deployed in an attempt to capture these often distinctly female domestic experiences, which feminists would later label as 'the problem that has no name'.[4] The analysis of MO and social science research in this chapter also points to the fundamental role that gendered household roles played in domestic tensions. Accounts of housework and the involvement, or lack of involvement, of husbands in such domestic work, foreground the conflicted nature of women's domestic roles, particularly the changing identity of the housewife in the post-war period, the shifting expectations of both work and leisure in the home and the contributory role of post-war housing shortages.

The Britain that emerged from the Second World War had become familiar with the centralised cultures of war, mobilisation and demo-bilisation and this enabled the development of a modern rationalised state that privileged planning, management and scientific methodolo-gies, among them sociological research, to address issues such as housing shortages and rebuilding. As Michael Savage has explained in his work on the development of social science in the post-war period, there was an increased focus on understanding and examining the everyday, on the practical and on eliciting direct responses from research subjects via interviews and questionnaires, which meant greater incursions into the lives of those who were the focus of government enquiry or other institutional research.[5] This chapter draws on several social scientific sources that used exactly these techniques to reveal the details of ordinary lives. However, these are illuminating not just for the detail they provide, but also in highlighting the sorts of subjects that govern-ment, industry, academia and individual researchers considered per-tinent at the time. For example, Hilda Brown's research in the mid-1950s into the effects of shift work was sponsored by the Ministry of Labour and National Service and intended to uncover the 'special social problems that arise from the introduction of multiple shifts' and to identify factors that affected worker attitudes to shifts. Such research was linked to the rise of multiple shift systems in factories but reflected concern about the effects on families as well as on shift-workers themselves. In doing so, such studies also revealed the unintended consequences, both positive and negative, of shift work for women's work within the home.[6] In examining the impact of changed work patterns, Brown's research was also examining the daily life of working-class families, and this professionalisation of areas of human experience which had previously been the private domain of individuals and families, arguably helped to frame a discourse which increasingly constituted everyday life as problematic, and paved the way for the evolution of stress as the explanation and expected response to such problems.

Such everyday troubles, including personal and intergenerational conflict, changing moral values and burgeoning consumerism, were reflected back to the population in popular culture of the late 1950s and early 1960s, and particularly in British New Wave films and television dramas. The interchange between the products of popular culture and the changing nature of both society and the media of popular culture itself in the post-war decades makes television and film valuable resources for understanding the ways in which experiences of domestic stress were both reproduced but also assimilated. The New Wave directors, Karl Reisz, John Schlesinger and Tony Richardson, were interested in extending the representation of the changing working classes and did so in a way which served both to 'reinforce and accelerate these changes' in films such as *Saturday Night and Sunday Morning*, *A Kind of Loving* and *The Loneliness of the Long Distance Runner*.[7] Their films portrayed versions of domestic life, class and housing that displayed a discontent and dissatisfaction that was apparently recognised and accepted by those audiences as representative of everyday life. With the majority of cinema-going audiences comprising young, working-class males in this period, such films offer insight into the male experience of domestic stress that is often missing from formal research into the domestic and illustrate emerging changes in social attitudes and behaviours through a medium that itself was changing and in its turn effecting social change.[8] The representation of working-class life that they offered, while not unproblematic, shows how the meanings of everyday domestic experience were being reflected and constituted at the time.[9] The cumulative effect of exposure to specific portrayals of such experience in popular culture was an influential factor in changing notions of gender roles, leisure, privacy, work and personal relationships, all of which contributed to a growing popular understanding that normalised domestic life as stressful.

Work in the home

Mrs C's account of her marriage serves as an example for a key cause of domestic stress; the relationship between husband and wife. Ali Haggett's interviews with women who were housewives in the 1950s and 1960s revealed that it was problems in their relationships much more than the nature of housewifery which led to the mental health problems they experienced.[10] While this chapter will nevertheless make the case for the contribution of housework to women's domestic stress, the role of interpersonal relationships was clearly critical. The experiences revealed in Mrs C's diaries bring to the fore issues about love, marriage, domestic roles, the use and control of time, space and family resources within the home, all of which contributed to one woman's self-reported mental breakdown. Her individual case is indicative of the complex interplay of factors which led to stress and unhappiness in many marriages, but which until the later twentieth century were often hidden and kept private from the outside world.

The diary that Mrs C kept and submitted to MO revealed a woman caught up in an unhappy marriage, trying to balance the demands of shift work as a nurse with childcare for her two daughters, the challenges of housekeeping, a secret love affair, and the jealousy and unpredictability of her conscripted husband Reg. Her accounts illustrate how often Reg thwarted her plans and disrupted her careful resource management and household planning. As Mrs C wrote in 1941, 'Been at home just 20 mins; when the trouble begins. Suggests that I had had my day off on Wed on purpose to avoid him. As if I could! Burns his dinner, which includes one person's meat ration for one week. Go to work heartbroken. I can't bear it any longer. I wonder what I'll do when the war is over? Went to bed in tears.'[11]

A common thread in the diary was the way in which Reg upset the careful balance of resources needed to run and maintain the home. For example, he insulted the next-door neighbour whom Mrs C relied on for childcare, so that she would not look after the children until he had gone back to the army.[12] His disruption of the niceties of the household's economics perhaps reflected the fact that managing the household budget and childcare were a wife's responsibilities, and therefore not his concern. The fact that his food and lodging were provided by the army when he was away from home might also have added to his lack of domestic awareness. However, it seems unlikely that he would have been completely oblivious to the difficulties of rationing or of the need for childcare, so it was not surprising that Mrs C complained,

> Fierce argument over lack of coal, sugar, tea and margarine. Told him straight that since he came home, we hadn't been able to save a crumb of anything towards Xmas. Ended in tears of sheer exasperation on my part! Had managed to save a bit of everything and had a cellar full of coal, last May – couldn't even close coal-cellar door. 6 months later, not a bit left, due to R's sheer callous extravagance!![13]

Although the responsibility for managing their resources might lie with the housewife, she was largely powerless to prevent others from squandering her efforts. It was the way in which the time and effort that she had put into managing those resources could be effectively negated by her husband that revealed to her the level of powerlessness in her situation. The inherent frustration and pointlessness of such a situation, in turn, caused Mrs C much stress and unhappiness.

The causes of domestic stress reflected the differing function of the home in the lives of men and women. For women, home was the location of their work, but also the heart of family life, while for men it was often their place of retreat from work. The home was understood as a desirable, domestic refuge, framed as both a physical location and psychological construct.[14] As scholars have argued, the meanings of home were multiple in this period and included ideas about material structure, permanence and continuity, security and control, refuge, status and family. The home might be a haven, a site of privacy and authenticity, and a shelter, with the relevance of any of these concepts depending on factors such as location, class, ethnicity and housing tenure.[15]

Women's accounts of their domestic relationships, and particularly the negotiation of roles and responsibilities within the home, illustrate

some of the key contributors to domestic stress. Examining the experience of the home from the housewife's perspective, along with analysing
attitudes towards their domestic role, reveals that the role itself brought
inherent tension through work which was largely unrewarding, unremit-
ting and often frustrating and boring: work could be a source of stress
in the home, as much as it could in paid employment. What was different
was that work outside the home could be validating through status
and social interaction, as discussed in Chapter 2, in a way that work
inside the home often was not.

In addition to the housewife role, how and whether women were
able to enjoy leisure was also a critical factor in domestic stress and
the role which husbands and families played was key to its amelioration
or exacerbation. In the immediate post-Second World War period there
were also underlying tensions in the fact that many middle-class women
were having to negotiate a different housewife identity from the pre-war,
servant-supported role they had been brought up to expect. There was
also a balance to be found between being a good enough housewife
and becoming a neurotic who was obsessively house-proud to the extent
that the home was no longer a home. For some women this was a
complex set of circumstances to negotiate successfully to their own
and their family's satisfaction, and for those unable to do so, a source
of considerable stress and anxiety.

As discussed in the previous chapter, many women had struggled
with the wartime burden of conscripted work and housework and
therefore it was unsurprising that many were all too keen to get back
to a solely domestic role after the war. As one woman told MO in 1944,
'The two jobs of home and work are getting me down. I'm tired.'[16] On
the other hand, for many women, working outside the home had been
their norm before the war and they expected it to be so afterwards.
As another told MO, 'I was here a long time before the war, and I'll
go on when it's over.'[17] Historians working on the effects of the Second
World War on women have contested the notion of war work as
emancipatory but pointed out that many women gained considerably
from their work through friendships, increased confidence and 'the
satisfaction of difficult work well done'.[18] Indeed, Mrs C reflected on
how her work as a nurse made her feel when commenting in her diary
on Reg's desire for her to give up her work: 'Have developed into a
Someone and at home I'd be a "NO-ONE".'[19] For Mrs C being a

housewife and mother was not a sufficiently satisfactory identity when she did not love her husband and it is impossible to know whether she would have felt differently if married to someone else. This is perhaps also reflected in the ambivalence of a twenty-year-old piece-worker who commented to MO, 'I don't want to stay on here myself, I wouldn't like to stay at home either, I'd get too bored.'[20] Undoubtedly such contradictions in women's experiences and attitudes also contributed towards the complexity of household dynamics in the post-war period.

Whether a woman continued to work outside the home after the war or not, what was indisputable was that she would most certainly be working inside the home. When housewives of the post-war period were asked in interviews whether they would have liked to have worked at this point in their lives, they responded with surprise, as in their minds, their domestic duties *were* work.[21] Somewhat unusually for the time, during the war Roffey Park Rehabilitation Centre had accepted housewives as industrial neurosis cases, suggesting a surprisingly progressive view of housework as work, or perhaps more likely, the influence of an expedient wartime ideology which conflated 'woman worker' with 'housewife', as Summerfield has argued.[22]

For working-class women, but also those of the middle classes who now found themselves servant-less and forced into the role of active housewife, the tension came partly from the conflicting nature of what the physical space of the home meant to its different inhabitants. Changing conceptions of the home resulting from the increasing expectations and aspirations of a steadily more affluent population after the Second World War were often the source of household tensions. This was not least because perceptions of what the home should be like (and particularly relationships within it) were often tinged with nostalgia or idealised in popular culture and individual aspirations, in a way that the reality of material circumstances could not match. Framing the home as a haven of belonging and security for men against the competition and challenges of the outside world of work ignored the fact that it could also be a location of unpaid, domestic labour and the locus of misery, anxiety and drudgery for women.[23] Home *was* predominantly a woman's workplace, while for the rest of the family, its main function was leisure. Thus, part of women's work in the home was about preserving that space of leisure and respite for the other members of the family.

An illustration of these tensions can be seen in research into the effects of shift work on domestic life carried out by Hilda Brown of the University of Sheffield in 1959 with funding from the Ministry of Labour and National Service. The research aimed to identify issues arising from the introduction of multiple shifts in five factories in the Midlands and North of England.[24] For Brown, 'The biggest complaint from the housewife was that she could not get on with her own work in the house if her husband was trying to sleep during the day ... the nervous strain caused by the necessity to keep quiet during the day was a serious hardship to some of the women.'[25] Brown's research involved interviews with 156 shift workers (and often their spouses) and was specifically focused on the social problems of shift working. She reported that one woman was so worried by the noise in the neighbourhood when her husband was trying to sleep that she could not get on with her work and went out of the house simply to keep out of the way. His shift work 'interfered both with her comfort and her peace of mind and [she] had become "nervy" and irritable'. Similarly, another woman's 'chief anxiety was in trying to keep the toddlers and baby quiet in the morning while her husband was sleeping', which meant that 'she also found it difficult to get her own housework done then'. The author reported that as a result both husband and wife 'felt irritable on this shift, and this caused friction at home'.[26] She also concluded, 'In view of the number of men who said they felt irritable or depressed when working at night, it is probable that more women felt the strain of an irritable husband in the home than admitted it.'[27] Not only was it a strain for the housewife to facilitate her husband's shift working, but she also had to accommodate his increased propensity to bad temper and irritability.

While shift work was not a new phenomenon, the Ministry of Labour and National Service had acknowledged as early as 1947 that industry was increasingly needful of longer working times to ensure economically efficient operations, and although not all organisations would require twenty-four hours of working, many would wish to adopt the double-day shift system.[28] While many workers would adapt to these changed patterns of work, evidently such adaptations could also contribute to new manifestations and articulations of stress, for wives and families as much as for male workers. Paradoxically, for women in paid employment, shift work could be perceived as beneficial in enabling them to carry two working roles more easily, greatly extending their working day, but also giving them more control through larger blocks of time at home. However, Brown's research also concluded that for female shift workers, 'The burden which it imposed on her as a wife and mother was the strain of being out at the times of day when her husband or family needed her most. The extent of this burden depended very much on the attitude of the husband.'[29] This was recognition that it was often factors outside of the housewife's control that had a significant effect on her mental well-being and an understanding spouse could make all the difference.

A husband's attitude was also revealed as pertinent in another study carried out by Judith Hubback among 1,500 women graduate and non-graduate wives in the 1950s. Hubback was a sociologist interested in married women's employment who carried out a self-funded postal survey of women graduates, initially published as a pamphlet by the Political and Economic Planning think-tank, but later expanded into a book.[30] She identified the issue of 'overtiredness', a condition she defined as 'when the person in question enjoys life much less than she usually does, wakes up tired or grows irritable early in the day, and looks and feels in every way far older than she is, all of this for more than a short time. There are other symptoms in plenty, varying with different people but the loss of enjoyment of life is the essential one.'[31] The description of 'loss of enjoyment of life' is recognisable from discussions of energy and fatigue that featured frequently in the self-help books examined in Chapter 1, and indeed tiredness was understood as both a cause and symptom of nervous conditions and tension from the early century onwards, appearing in industrial and military research as well as popular self-help.[32] While we might now also understand Hubback's description as possibly representing symptoms of depression, her use of 'overtiredness' suggests a euphemism that was perhaps more acceptable to her research subjects than nerves, stress or depression might have been, suggesting as it did a physical problem. Hubback's questionnaire asked participants both about the causes of overtiredness, but also the causes of *not* feeling overtired. For 36 per cent of graduate wives and 27 per cent of non-graduate wives, helpful husbands were a key factor in not feeling overtired. For the former this constituted the highest-scoring factor and for the latter was beaten only by 'good health'. Hubback concluded that it was not straining the figures too far to state that a cooperative husband was a key factor in housewives avoiding 'overtiredness'.[33]

Unfortunately, as with Mrs C and Reg, not many husbands seemed to realise this. The following remark from one man responding to MO's research in 1943 on psychological factors in home-building illustrates a blithe unconcern: 'I am convinced that my home will never be a showpiece. For though my wife if given her time, will bring up everything to a spotless condition, the children and I will soon muck it up again.'[34] His comment highlights two critical factors: it acknowledges the husband's contribution to the endless cycle of housework and it refers to the idea of the home as a showpiece, suggesting this was a desirable goal. His dismissive comment implies that having a 'spotless' home was not his ambition, but instead the seemingly futile goal of his wife's endless labour. Some women did derive satisfaction from housework, not as a process but in terms of the resulting product. Thus one explained to MO in a 1951 survey on housework, 'though I dislike most of the jobs singly, collectively I derive satisfaction from housework because I have a nice home which rewards me with its beauty when cleaned'. Most pertinently, she also pointed out that 'I could not get this same satisfaction were I poor and my possessions tawdry and ugly.'[35] She made a clear link between housework and a 'nice home' which explicitly involved the evidence of consumption through the display of material possessions.

For others, such as a primary school teacher, that sort of pride in the result of such tedious daily work meant 'they are likely to become obsessed with tidiness and cleanliness so that they become most unpleasant people with whom to live and their home is only a house'.[36] This teacher's comments expressed revulsion at the idea of the home being nothing more than a way of projecting a story of external display. Here again was the concern seen earlier in self-help books that women could become obsessed with their homes, and that such an obsession could make them neurotic, although this time it was a woman expressing the view. A young man summed it up in explaining to MO that a housewife 'must not put her house before her home, becoming house-proud'.[37] To be house-proud was a negative quality because this was pride in the material and that was not apparently what constituted a home. Such an interpretation also suggested that the housewife had to find the point of balance between being an efficient housewife and becoming obsessed. The negative connotations of being house-proud are also interesting in that to some extent they denied women the natural outcome of working hard. Effectively finding purpose in what was often a rather purposeless set of activities was wrong because it somehow impinged on the idea of home as a place of relaxation and retreat. That men and women might have contradictory ideals of the home because it signified something different (for him a retreat, for her the product of her labour) would almost inevitably provide the potential for conflict, tension and frustration.

Help for housewives

Some of that tension and frustration was starting, by the late 1940s and early 1950s, to be aired publicly and nationally, recognised by government and reflected in media coverage. This placed the issue of how domestic work and household duties could affect the mental health of housewives beyond simply a medical discussion as had occurred with the identification of suburban neurosis in the 1930s and into a much wider and more accessible popular discourse. This was partly due to the efforts of some of the middle-class women who found themselves struggling in the post-war period to maintain homes designed for a time before the servant class had all but disappeared into more lucrative and less exhausting work elsewhere.[38] Although the reduction in domestic help was part of a long-term trend, exacerbated by the war, it was recognised as early as 1944 as a potentially serious post-war problem. Research for the Ministry of Labour and National Service into planning for post-war domestic employment acknowledged that among those women who had previously had domestic servants, there was already 'much evidence of strain and consequent ill-health' during wartime, but could offer little in the way of planned post-war help, beyond proposals to professionalise domestic service through training and improved pay.[39] Further evidence of the prominence given to the issue can be seen in a discussion on the BBC in 1946 entitled *Help for Housewives*.[40] Arguably, the programme demonstrated attempts to salvage some class distinctions from a situation in which a middle-class housewife carried much the same burden as a working-class one, by focusing on the more genteel elements of housework such as sewing, decorating and cooking, which were more aligned to middle-class aspirations.[41] Such attempts were one way for middle-class women to reconcile themselves to their new housewife identity in a manner which maintained class differences.

Although for much of the twentieth century women's experiences of domestic stress had been largely hidden behind closed doors and not discussed, partly because of a reluctance to conceptualise the home and domestic life as problematic and partly because of mores relating to privacy, this changed in the post-war period.[42] The problems of housewifery and the effects of housework on women were still garnering public interest nearly ten years after the BBC broadcast in a series of letters from middle-class housewives in the *Manchester Guardian* newspaper in October 1954, prompted by an initial letter from Margaret Hughes. She wrote to the editor,

> For some time I have been seriously disturbed at the great strain under which we wives are living in these new housing estates with – as one would think – every modern convenience physically, and every emotional satisfaction, of a husband and young children just at their most endearing age. Two or three of my acquaintances are having mental treatment and almost every household nearby runs by a series of crises due to temporary minor collapses of the wife.[43]

She went on to mention the 'great strain of never being off duty' while other letters referred to acquaintances 'nervy with neurotic cleaning and polishing' who 'couldn't leave the housework'.[44] Another correspondent suggested that housewives should 'develop one or two outside interests – the best counterbalance to nervous strain brought on by inflexible devotion to household tasks', which was notably similar to self-help book advice, discussed in Chapter 1.[45] However, other women wrote in to argue different causes and solutions. According to Mrs Saunders, the nub of the problem was that a husband and young children did not offer emotional satisfaction as claimed by Mrs Hughes: 'So many modern men tied to an office desk or factory bench for six days a week, quite voluntarily doing overtime in many cases, are far too emotionally restless to be anything but a source of aggravation to their wives.' In fact, she believed that it was 'rash in the extreme to assume that fathers have begun sharing much of the work of the home'.[46] Another housewife proposed that material consumption (or at least the desire for it) combined with the current age of 'insecurity and instability' was a greater cause of women's woes than 'having too much to do and being too much in non-adult company'.[47] After a week or so of such published debate, the *Manchester Guardian* editor closed the correspondence, presumably worried that it would run and run. The fact that Mrs Hughes's original letter garnered such a response (and that the newspaper chose to publish the correspondence) was indicative of the unresolved debate over the expectations, perceived role and actual experience of housewives, and reflected an increasing recognition and articulation of domestic stress.

This debate was effectively part of a wider discourse about the nature of marriage itself, focused particularly on the concept of the companionate marriage which carried with it a range of ideas, including marriage as teamwork, marriage based on sharing and companionship, and on partnership and equality. These ideas were also part of deliberations on marriage at state level, which included a Royal Commission on Marriage and Divorce in 1956, but which settled on encouraging adjustments to marital expectations as a way of adapting to changing social mores, rather than the enactment of more liberal divorce legislation.[48] However, the ideas behind companionate marriage, as the letters to the *Manchester Guardian* show, were not necessarily realised, particularly regarding equality of domestic responsibilities. As Mrs C's case shows, Reg played no part in the management of the household and in some instances appeared to deliberately disrupt her careful planning by wasting scarce rationed food and alienating her source of childcare. Their apparently different expectations of marriage and understandings of marital responsibilities were reflected in a complaint she made in 1944 about the material condition of her home: 'Sat with my head resting in my hands too full for words – too full to cry even but desperately fed-up. Look around at old rugs, old walls, gaslight and think bitterly of all the money R has lost in the past.'[49] Mrs C undoubtedly blamed Reg for the condition of their furnishings and fittings, because he had apparently squandered money. Yet she was working and earning money so was potentially able to contribute to the cost of replacing some of these items. What this suggests is the strength of accepted gendered domestic responsibilities within the household; breadwinning for men and housekeeping for women, with no apparent deviation possible.[50] Finch and Summerfield have argued that rather than being of benefit to women, ideas about companionate marriage simply created contradictory pressures which placed greater strain on women and pushed them towards a type of marriage which 'made extra demands without necessarily providing extra rewards'.[51] Thus, even if Mrs C's had been more of a companionate marriage, the suggestion is that this would not have solved her problems.

There was a paradox at play in terms of the domestic space: on the one hand this was the female domain for which the housewife was almost totally responsible, and yet on the other, her control of the space and of her time within it were ultimately subject to others who could, albeit often unwittingly, within a short period nullify the work of many hours, and the planned activities of many more. As a result, many women found themselves bound to the home in a relentless effort to keep on top of their domestic role, with the concomitant stress and strain that this created, often articulated as tiredness and nervous collapse: a phenomenon that was not lost on researchers still pursuing the concept of suburban neurosis. What was significant about this was that it was becoming more visible within a public discourse that encompassed women's roles as wife, mother and worker.

Suburban neurosis revisited

It is notable that in Mrs Hughes's original letter to the *Manchester Guardian* she referred to the strain on wives living on 'new housing estates'.[52] In the post-war period, there was a desperate need for new housing as well as a continuation of the interwar drive to replace slum housing, both of which accelerated the creation of more suburban estates. However, concerns remained amongst those responsible for planning new estates and new towns about the potentially deleterious effects of suburban living with planners determined to create environments which would avoid the problem of suburban neurosis. As a result, considerable research was undertaken by public health experts both in the immediate post-war period to further understand the problem, and in the new towns and estates themselves, once they were built, in the hope of proving that the problem had been overcome. Such research undoubtedly contributed to the increasing process of problematising aspects of everyday life that might previously have been either ignored or kept private. At the same time, concerns about suburban neurosis reflected ongoing class-based assumptions and snobberies about suburbs and new towns, where most residents were working-class, but also the aspirations of post-war generations determined to build a better Britain.[53]

Between 1946 and 1950 eleven new towns were designated in England, including Harlow and Crawley.[54] A 1958 editorial in *The Lancet* reported that 'In the new towns, industry and homes have moved out together, imaginative social provision has done much to reduce the risk of neurotic reactions in a new environment.' However, 'out-county, municipal estates' were suspected of repeating the pre-war problems and *The Lancet* reported research by the London School of Hygiene and Tropical Medicine (LSHTM), which appeared to show that suburban neurosis was 'presenting itself again'. On one new estate admissions to mental hospitals between 1949 and 1954 were more than 50 per cent above what would be expected from national figures, with 'neurotic reactive depression among females predominating'. Information from GPs showed that the self-estimate of nerves on one estate was 223 per 1,000 adults, compared with a national figure of 126. Complaints of neurotic symptoms were higher among those who had lived on the estate for less than two years than among those whose occupancy dated back over three years. The conclusion drawn was that 'Physical planning on the out-county estates appears to be out of step with social planning and rehousing has improved physical environment at the cost of mental wellbeing.'[55]

One large-scale research project was undertaken by Sidney Chave from the LSHTM into the new town of Harlow, which had been designed specifically to counter suburban neurosis. As one of the researchers explained in the mid-1960s,

> There is a commonly held view that the housing estates create conditions which are conducive to the development of neurosis. This is said to arise from the strains consequent upon removal from a familiar to an unfamiliar area, in which ties with home and kin are attenuated or even severed altogether. The social isolation combined with the financial stresses arising from the move have been said to provide the predisposing conditions for worry, anxiety and sometimes for frank neurosis, especially among young housewives.[56]

This view was one which permeated much thinking in the late 1950s and early 1960s, and was subsequently repeated by sociologists and historians alike, reinforced by work such as *Family and Kinship in East*

London, which studied the effects of slum clearance rehousing policy on a close-knit community.[57] However, the results of the Harlow research were surprising: there were fewer cases of mental illness receiving in-patient treatment from Harlow than was expected compared to the experience of the general population; the prevalence of anxiety and tension states reported by GPs was not highest among young housewives, but among women aged 45 to 54, that is menopausal women; and a comparison of those with nerves and those without could show no important variable among factors such as length of residence, income or extent of their contacts with relations and friends living outside Harlow. The only significant difference for this group was that they 'had made fewer friends, participated less in community activities, were more beset with problems, and expressed greater dissatisfaction with the town than the rest'.[58]

That it was not necessarily the geographical location that was the problem for this cohort of women was something that one of the few female self-help authors mentioned in Chapter 1, Flora Klickmann, had explained forty years earlier in 1925:

> While a woman's life is fully occupied with her children and household, or with business responsibilities, she has not the time to brood over little discomforts or small troubles. It is when her children no longer need her, when the home requires but little supervision from her, or when circumstances of one sort or another have cut her off from the running activities of life, that she suddenly finds the hours drag and realises that she no longer has the physical elasticity that would enable her to embark on new ventures or a round of excitements.[59]

Klickmann's description of what became known as empty-nest syndrome seems a much more likely explanation for the distress of this group of women, suggesting issues that were specific to their age, their life experiences and their changing roles, rather than the location of their home. Based on the Harlow findings and others, the LSHTM researchers were forced to admit that this was not suburban neurosis, and instead concluded that 'these are the people who carry their neurosis with them wherever they go and project their inner disharmony upon their environment'. Such people could be found anywhere, and 'the people of the new town differed but little from those living in and around the metropolitan city which had once been their home'.[60]

Despite these conclusions, the idea of a specifically suburban neurosis was remarkably persistent, with further research carried out in Bristol in the 1970s, where apparently the problem of neurosis among women was reaching 'very high levels in suburban locations'.[61] The research was part of a wider programme, the Gulbenkian Housing Research Project, conducted by the Department of Mental Health at Bristol University, and funded by the Calouste Gulbenkian Foundation. Unsurprisingly it found no more conclusive answers than the earlier research. It suggested that concern about social status might be a contributing factor but also that while some wives 'gave familiar accounts of feelings of suburban boredom, or the frustration of lonely days in the company only of their young children, others complained of the tightness of family budgeting which obliged them to go out to work for extra money'.[62] All that the research had proved was that although the environment could provide a focus for sufferers to project their unhappy feelings, it was not necessarily the cause of them.[63] The causes were largely within the home and complex dynamics of family life, not least women's often limited opportunities for leisure.

Women's leisure

As we saw in Chapter 1, Flora Klickmann identified one of the problems of the housewife role in her 1925 self-help book *Mending Your Nerves*, when she pointed out that unlike other roles, the hours were not fixed and the housewife's responsibilities always with her.[64] In essence, it was the gendered nature of the female domestic roles, and particularly their wider caring responsibilities, that were often at the root of their stress. She had also recommended that women have at least an hour a day to themselves, and recommended even simple breaks such as taking a bus journey out of town.[65] The point being made in all the self-help books of the interwar period was that overtaxing the system was detrimental to mental as well as physical health and that one way of avoiding this was to spend time doing things that were enjoyable, such as hobbies. Self-help books of the mid-century similarly endorsed this point, with a BMA publication, *How to Live With Your Nerves and Like It*, suggesting, 'Going to the pictures can be a good emotional purge – the Epsom salts of the emotions. I find if you're not too depressed – just anxious and tense and fed-up – that a sad picture makes you feel as happy as a sand boy when you leave the theatre. But a good funny picture can do the trick too.'[66] The continuity of this advice suggests that for many women, little had changed in the intervening decades, in terms of their control of time and any recognition of their need for leisure. Often even these simple remedies were unachievable, giving them little opportunity to alleviate the strains of domestic life.

Research by MO in 1945 into the reasons people gave for having small families reported that 'More women mentioned loss of freedom and extra work as an unforeseen snag of married life than any other item.'[67] Conflicting attitudes towards use of time and control of domestic activities were not uncommon, as Hannah Gavron found when carrying out interviews with 96 middle- and working-class housewives in London nearly twenty years later as part of her PhD research.[68] Her work aimed to understand their experiences as housewives and particularly any conflict they experienced as a result of their role. One working-class housewife told Gavron, 'The trouble is when he comes home in the evenings all he wants to do is watch television, he's tired, you see. Whereas for me, well I've been home all day and I'd like to go out.'[69] Her comments illustrate differing conceptualisations of home: for him, it was a haven of rest and relaxation, but for her, it was a workplace and therefore relaxation came from leaving it. Gavron's research found that in fact 31 per cent of the working-class couples in her survey never went out in the evenings. Some women without babysitting arrangements let their husbands go out without them, which meant that 44 per cent of these mothers never went out in the evening at all. Of the 56 per cent who could go out only half of them did so regularly once a week compared with two-thirds of Gavron's middle-class sample.[70] The title of Gavron's book, *The Captive Wife*, was revealing of her interpretation of her findings. Many women's lives were contained in a way that allowed little release for any tensions that arose within the home.

Gavron's research noted that since the Second World War there had been a reduction in the age at marriage so that by 1960 more than a quarter of all brides were under twenty.[71] This partly explained the rueful tone of some of her interviewees, such as one working-class woman who told her, 'It's feeling so stuck what with the kids and everything', while another commented, 'Even if you've had your fling it doesn't make up for this tied down feeling.'[72] This might also be compounded by spousal attitudes, as a husband in Wigan responding to a MO survey in 1949, demonstrated: 'My wife I haven't much time for. I don't have time to take her out.'[73] In the post-war decades, the norm was for many housewives to spend most of their time in the home, going out in the evening only rarely. Their ability to escape the home was largely outside of their control, being mediated by the attitudes of husbands, particularly their willingness to care for children, but also their acceptance of their wife's need for external leisure. That there might be little awareness of such a need was linked to conceptual understandings of leisure which saw it as something earned through full-time labour. Even with the increased participation of married women in the workforce as part-time or casual labour, this was often denied them because combining housework with a part-time job was not perceived as 'deserving of a leisure reward'.[74] However, the very nature of Gavron's research, focusing as it did on ordinary women's lives and the constraints on them, demonstrates once again the increasing exposure of what had previously been private, and with it the problematising of aspects of domestic life that contributed to women's stress. Exacerbating such problems for those not living in new towns or estates was the dire shortage of housing. For while life on new housing estates could create its own form of stress, so could the forced family togetherness of those not lucky enough to enjoy new homes.

Overcrowding and the struggle for privacy

Post-war Britain had a huge housing problem. The slum clearances and estate building of the 1920s and 1930s had been halted by the war, but the housing problems they had tried to address continued, compounded now by wartime damage and destruction. While five million demobbed servicemen and women were only too glad to have returned home, the difference between the imagined home of their wartime separation and the experience of the people and place they found on their return was sometimes considerable, as was the impact of their homecoming on the family they had left behind.[75] Thus, the practical disruptions of war also brought with them conceptual ones, as ideas about what home was and how family relationships might work were revisited, resolved or revealed as a source of conflict, as seen in the case of Mrs C and Reg. The housing situation of the post-war period brought to light the psychological as well as the physical problems that arose from overcrowding and intergenerational conflict and made them more public.

Despite the problems of life on the interwar county estates and urban slums, those who did manage to get a house or even a flat in such areas were among the lucky, for if housing provision had been problematic before the Second World War, it was dramatically worse afterwards. As MO reported in 1945 in a survey on women's reasons for having small families, 'Next to money, housing was the most frequently mentioned deterrent to having children. There were many comments on the difficulty of finding anywhere to live, particularly from the newly married who were often living with their parents under overcrowded conditions.'[76] A further MO report on the state of matrimony published two years later based on a survey in eight London boroughs and Gloucester, showed that of those married five years or less, 56 per cent were living with relatives. For those married between five and ten years, a fifth were still doing so, and for those married more than ten years, 10 per cent were still living with relatives.[77] Other surveys supported this picture of limited housing provision, overcrowding and poor conditions.[78]

One young woman interviewed by MO gave such tensions as her main reason when asked why she wanted to get married. 'To get out of my Mum's house more than anything. My Mum and Dad were always squabbling; he's fond of his pint, and he used to have more than was good for him, and that used to set them off. I wanted to get married and have a home of my own and a bit of peace.'[79] A 1949 social survey carried out for the Ministry of Health, looking at the housing conditions of people on local authority housing waiting lists, found that 46 per cent gave their reason for wanting to move as overcrowding, 26 per cent as wanting a home of their own and 18 per cent on grounds of health.[80] Research into changing marriage habits carried out ten years later as part of the Population Investigation Committee's Survey, found little difference: asked about 'marriage adjustment problems', a sample of 3,000 men and women, interviewed in 1959–1960, reported housing at the top of their list. One couple's typical experience was explained: 'marrying in April 1957 when the groom was 21 and the bride only 16, with a baby on the way, lived first with one lot of parents and then the other until their second child was born in January 1959, when they obtained furnished rooms ... this couple listed housing as the main problem, but both parents and in-laws as additional difficulties'.[81] The conclusion of the research analysis while clarifying that housing problems led to a breakdown in marriage in only a few cases, established that 'the distress caused by inadequate housing was widespread'.[82] Housing was undoubtedly the main issue, the effects of short supply resulting in strain on family relationships due to sharing facilities, but also conflict over control of resources and domestic roles.[83] That issue of control was increasingly fuelled by the differing values and expectations of the post-war generation and their parents, values that were in part a result of the burgeoning consumer culture that increasingly intruded into domestic life via the television and other forms of popular culture.

Domestic tensions and kitchen-sink dramas

By 1960 the problems of intergenerational living and housing shortages were becoming very visible in popular culture. Television ownership had spread rapidly during the 1950s so that by 1963, 82 per cent of households had a television, enabling them to enjoy the common culture it was both reflecting and creating.[84] Starting in 1956 and broadcast in the Sunday evening slot for almost twenty years, the weekly *Armchair Theatre* drama anthology on the Independent Television (ITV) channel offered single performances which, according to their producer Sydney Newman, were intended to reflect contemporary change, not the 'dated West End plays' which perpetuated the old class-based society.[85] He told *The Observer* that one of the 'cardinal tenets of my thinking is the dynamic change which is taking place in Britain: it is these changing relationships that must be the subject matter for a good TV play'.[86] Indeed, he was open about his intent to dramatise the 'problems of an increasing materialism' but also to reflect how the 'manners and mores' of his twenty-one million television viewers were changing in response to their viewing.[87] What Newman's view, unsurprisingly for a television enthusiast, did not acknowledge was the way in which viewing his product might change the dynamics within the home and alter the experience of everyday domesticity. The huge growth in television viewing in the late 1950s meant that the location of much leisure was shifting from outside the home to inside it. The implications of such a shift might, on the one hand, be interpreted as positive for increasing the focus on the family taking their leisure together, but equally such a shift might also simply exacerbate any existing domestic discord through such togetherness, and once again deny women the possibility of external leisure.[88]

The ongoing tensions of intergenerational living and the gendered nature of caring responsibilities were played back through a 1960 episode of *Armchair Theatre* entitled 'Where I live', which dramatised the family conflict caused by a brother and sister battling over which one was to house their widowed father.[89] In one scene, Jessy, the sister, is seen washing the dishes and her father approaches to help, but she rebuffs him, telling him to 'sit down and keep quiet' and to 'go and read your paper in the lounge'. It is evident from her curt dealings with him that she simply does not want him around, even though he is clearly looking for company. He goes in search of the cat in the yard, and she stops him, saying, 'I don't want him under my feet all the time when I'm trying to work', a sentiment which is evidently directed at her father as much as the cat. The 'dynamic change' that Newman talked about was one in which the intergenerational living that had been the norm for many of the poorest working-class families for years, was now unacceptable to members of a more aspirational consumer culture. Jessy's apparently sudden decision that her brother should take his turn in offering a home to their father is indicative of her changing expectations of her role as daughter, sister and housewife. The conflict that this creates only adds to the stress that she has been experiencing as she is torn between the societal norms of female caring responsibilities and her own desire for respite and to live a different sort of life.[90]

Another source of British social realism presenting the issues of the day, and also defined by opposition to middle-class comedies and dramas, were the films of the so-called British 'New Wave', such as *A Kind of Loving*, *Saturday Night and Sunday Morning* and *The Loneliness of the Long Distance Runner*.[91] Winning multiple film awards in Britain and abroad and featuring among the most popular releases of the early 1960s, these productions were, according to the *Daily Mirror*, 'raw, earthy and bursting with a vital, provincial realism'.[92] They were also all 'X' rated by the British Board of Film Classification, a factor which perhaps proved useful in promoting their popularity amongst the young working-class men who now made up the majority of the cinema-going audience.[93] It has been argued that these films were 'pioneering', depicting their subject matter 'more intently and more realistically than any British motion pictures had done to that time', and being positively received as a result of this honesty.[94] While there is now debate as to just how far they can be seen as a 'force for progressive change in society', nevertheless they were clear in their criticism of some of the 'reticent conventions of British society', and showed that change was taking place at the time.[95] Such 'reticent conventions' included the strong sense of privacy about domestic difficulties that restricted women like Mrs C to her MO writings and led middle-class housewives to jump at the chance of acknowledgement and discussion of the difficulties they were experiencing in the *Manchester Guardian* in the mid-1950s.

While acknowledging that these films were by no means the first representations in feature films of the condition of the working classes, what they did do was ensure that class differences were 'unambiguous and explicit'.[96] It was precisely because they centred on the lives of the industrial working classes that at the time they were acclaimed for offering greater authenticity than previous representations. Arguably, the films can be seen as middle-class interpretations of the realities of life for the working classes precisely because by focusing on the personal they avoided the economic and industrial issues which underpinned many of the social problems portrayed.[97] However, according to one contemporary critic, writing in *The Times*, 'the new directors are showing us ... aspects of England we have never been shown before'.[98] Apparently so convincing were the problems portrayed, that two Labour MPs arranged for a special screening of *A Kind of Loving* in the House of Commons because they believed it 'spotlights the housing problem better than any documentary'.[99]

What the films depicted was a domestic life characterised by intergenerational conflict, divided social aspirations, contradictory ideals and the tensions of insufficient privacy. It showed young people constrained physically by the lack of housing and mentally by the knowledge that there were no quick solutions, and provided a male perspective on such domestic strain, through their leading protagonists. They also illuminated the everyday aggravation of constant compromises to enable some sort of modus operandi, all of which pointed to a high level of domestic stress, which nevertheless was rarely articulated. A further contribution to such tensions was suggested by the increasing visibility of idealised versions of the home delivered to people who could scarcely envisage let alone afford them, via the medium of television, in both programming and advertisements.

The mostly middle-class occupants of Westminster watching the special screening may not have seen this England before, but the cinema-going population at which the films were aimed surely had. That population was young, male and working-class, the traditional family audience having mostly transferred its allegiance to television by the early 1960s.[100] If the authenticity of films comes less from portraying convincing details, and more from presenting a narrative which viewers perceived as a true picture of life showing a plausible universe consonant with their values and attitudes, then the popularity of these films with the regular cinema-going population of young men would seem to confirm that they found in them a fair reflection of their own lives.[101] Certainly, the main protagonists were young males, and it was their problematic relationships with family and women, and the stress arising from them, that were being explored in a way that reflected a construction of young working-class masculinity as tough, cynical, irresponsible, self-centred and underpinned by a culture of hedonism.[102] While some historians have argued that the contemporary concerns about inter-generational conflict were overstated and that many working-class parents celebrated the opportunities that the economic security of the time offered their children, it was also the case that many of those parents still adhered to traditional social values, which meant their aspirations were somewhat at odds with those of their children.[103]

One example of conflicting parental aspirations, housing shortage and intergenerational tension leading to stress can be seen in A Kind of Loving, released in 1962, where the leading character, Vic, moves into his mother-in-law's house after a shotgun marriage to his pregnant on/off girlfriend, Ingrid. The Britain in which the film was set was still a country in which the institution of marriage was broadly supported, but the questions it raised about the nature of gender, family and domestic relations highlight the level of contemporary anxiety about these issues.[104] As one critic identified, part of the conflict portrayed came from tensions around class and social mobility, with Vic enduring the 'wailings of his mother-in-law about the class of various competitors who appear on her favourite zombie television quiz shows'.[105] Tension arose from the conflicting aspirations of different generations. Thus, in *A Kind of Loving*, Vic's mother-in-law is shown to be disappointed in her daughter's marriage as she perceives herself and Ingrid to be socially superior, evidenced through the location, size and style of their semi-detached house and their conspicuous material consumption. Vic comes from a traditional, terraced, back-to-back house, his father working for the railway and his mother seen scrubbing the front step. They represent the traditional working classes, whereas his mother-in-law with her aspirations and consumerism represents the worst side of the new affluence.[106]

A similar theme can be seen in *Saturday Night and Sunday Morning*, released in 1960, where the lead character, Arthur Seaton, rejects his own parents' passive acceptance of their lot in the same back-to-back terraces, where neighbours bicker and interfere in each other's lives: 'They've got a television set and a packet of fags but they're dead from the neck up', he claims.[107] Both Vic and Arthur are portrayed as wanting more from life, but both are trapped by circumstances, living in houses with parents or in-laws with different values and expectations of them. That they will fail to escape and instead perpetuate this limited existence is the ultimate message of both films: Vic because he must live in poor and degrading housing in order to escape his mother-in-law's home and rescue his marriage, and Arthur because his upwardly mobile girlfriend has clear ambitions for a house on a new estate outside Nottingham that she can furnish with new goods, which he will have to work to pay for. Much of the tension in the protagonists' relationships with their partners and families is portrayed as coming from this inherent knowledge. The characters are portrayed as attempting to rebel against their circumstances, but the apparent futility of such rebellion is also contributory to the stressful nature of their lives.

In another film of the period, *The Loneliness of the Long Distance Runner*, released in 1962, the lead character Colin Smith's home is in a pre-fab with his dying father and a mother impatient for his life insurance money. Her focus on material consumption is underlined by the large television she buys, which is mocked by Colin and his friends but holds the rest of the family in thrall. Her rush to purchase consumer goods might be seen as an attempt to create the kind of home she has previously seen portrayed on other people's televisions and at a cinema which up to that point had tended more to domestic idealisation than the gritty realities of the so-called kitchen-sink drama.[108] But her rapid spending of money which, it is hinted, she received by prematurely hastening her husband's death, simply serves to highlight how unlike the idealised home of popular culture her shabby and crowded pre-fab is. The television looms large over a room where nobody speaks, and Colin is left to his own devices, ultimately ending up in borstal and his case proving unequivocally that television did not necessarily promote the family togetherness that the discourse of advertising and new technology might suggest.[109]

All three films feature television as a symbol of increasing consumerism, particularly among the working classes of the period, with their growing disposable income. However, television can also be seen to prompt a passivity which accepted the existing class and economic structure and perhaps even protected against the inherent tensions of the home. Without the rooms to enable physical privacy, people escaped conflict by sitting silently in front of the television, switched off from human interaction. In *A Kind of Loving*, Vic's mother-in-law's commentary on the class of the participants in quiz shows fortified her own class prejudices, subtly reinforcing the difference she perceived between Vic and Ingrid, while in *Saturday Night and Sunday Morning* Arthur Seaton's father's mindless viewing served to block out the reality of his dreary existence and annoying neighbours. To some extent, television therefore becomes a tool that can both produce stress, in Vic's experience of his mother-in-law's prejudices, or supress and avoid it, in the case of his father. That film-makers portrayed television in a negative light is not altogether surprising when, between 1955 and 1960, cinema was experiencing a rapid audience decline and television a massive growth.[110] However, despite any self-serving interest, their portrayal highlights some of the tensions and inadequacies of homes that did not fulfil their idealised function as places of comfort, love and privacy.

The latter is the key to the tensions in Vic and Ingrid's married life in *A Kind of Loving*, as living in her mother's house means living by her rules and with her constant interference. Despite being working adults, the lead characters must live like children because of the shortage of housing. As Marwick noted, this must have rung true with many young people in cinema audiences at the time and it was certainly consistent with government research into housing waiting lists discussed earlier.[111] However, even their parents struggle, as Arthur's father, in *Saturday Night and Sunday Morning*, is portrayed suffering the intrusion of the nosey and complaining neighbours who make up the tightly packed community in the terraced streets. The feuding, bickering neighbourhood illustrated would no doubt have been familiar to the MO correspondent mentioned in Chapter 2, who bemoaned the lack of fights on her new estate.[112] For him, it is a source of aggravation and stress and something to escape from through mindless television watching.

In many ways, the central characteristic of the British New Wave films was the fragility of families and the identification of home as a space of conflict and anxiety that normalised the idea of domestic stress.[113] The representation of the domestic life of working-class people offered a much more troubled and contested space than the post-war discourse of domesticity might have suggested.[114] Both film and television drama were reflecting changes in society through the portrayal of intergenerational conflict, the effects of consumerist expectations and the changing values and morality of the post-war generation. At the same time, popular culture itself was changing with leisure consumption shifting noticeably inside the home through the massively increased audience for television. This shift in itself might also be interpreted as contributing to the very domestic stresses it was representing on screen: first because it brought people together around the television within the contested space of the home, rather than providing a breathing space through external leisure activities; second through its promulgation of idealisations of everyday life which played a significant role in driving the consumer and social aspirations which in many cases were also at the heart of domestic conflict; and third, when it did represent the discontents, unhappy compromises and frustrations of domestic experience, in dramas such as the *Armchair Theatre* series, by confirming and thus validating such negative experiences without necessarily offering any useful solutions. Ultimately what popular culture offered was the normalisation of the idea that domestic life was stressful.

Conclusion

Mrs C's unhappy marriage, as described by her to MO, provides an insight into the stress arising from personal relationships, particularly in relation to issues of control of time and resources and the impact of a husband's actions on workload and domestic planning. Her diaries and handful of letters to MO referred to strain and in one case to a 'mental breakdown', although she provided few details.[115] While the label 'stress' was not yet in common usage to describe such experiences, the experiences themselves *were* common. This was apparent from housewives' letters to the *Manchester Guardian* detailing their experiences of nerves, as well as from the responses to researchers such as Brown, Gavron and Hubback, that identified the nature of housework and the role of husbands and children in creating a never-ending workload as contributing to domestic strain and 'tiredness'. At the heart of this was the contested nature of the home: for men a refuge from work and the outside world but for many women the main location of their labour, and a labour that was not necessarily recognised as such by others.

One interpretation of female responses to such situations was the persistent concept of suburban neurosis: an idea that informed much post-war new town and estate building, but which was also ultimately undermined and discredited when research in post-war estates and new towns failed to substantiate its claims regarding causation, despite the continuing existence of the underlying problems it encapsulated. Such research was pertinent in reflecting the increased incursion of experts into the domestic realm in the post-war period. Although the interest in suburban neurosis was grounded in a post-war desire to improve the living conditions of ordinary people, it was also indicative of the professionalisation of areas of human experience that had previously been private. The interest of experts in the daily existence of the populace helped to frame a discourse that increasingly constituted everyday life as problematic, encouraging the articulation of nervous troubles and paving the way for the evolution of stress as the explanation and response to such problems.

In the accounts women gave of their domestic experiences to MO and in various research projects, two parallel threads emerge that tie their work to stress: on the one hand the repetitive nature of housework, the need for it endlessly renewed by everyday family life that made for frustration, drudgery and a never-ending attempt to wrest control; on the other, the risk of both housework and increasing consumerism and materialism driving the housewife to extremes of neuroticism and a negatively perceived focus on being house-proud. The very fact that there was public debate in a national newspaper and government involvement in broadcasting about this issue suggests that the extent of its impact was widely and publicly recognised. It was not only the Sisyphean nature of housewifery that created domestic tension, but often the very nature of how people lived, particularly as a result of the housing shortages that lasted well beyond the immediate post-war period. Such shortages meant many people lived in overcrowded homes, creating tensions over use and control of resources. This was particularly the case for newly-wed couples, many of whom lived with parents or in-laws for several years. Such situations were increasingly reflected in popular culture and both television dramas and mass-market films dramatised interpersonal and intergenerational strain. Not only did they reflect such strain, arguably they also helped fuel it. A growing consumer culture offered aspirational images of ideal homes, and it was often the clash of values between the aspirations of the post-war generation and their parents that aggravated domestic stress. It was that same post-war generation who were also to become the focus of a more general popular discourse about stress and everyday life in the latter decades of the twentieth century.

Notes

1 D5284, 'Letter to Mass Observation', 4 March 1942, MOA, University of Sussex.
2 D5284, 'Letter to Mass Observation', 4 February 1943, MOA, University of Sussex.
3 *Ibid.*
4 Betty Friedan, *The Feminine Mystique* (London: Penguin, 1965), p. 13.
5 Michael Savage, *Identities and Social Change in Britain since 1940: The Politics of Method* (Oxford: Oxford University Press, 2010), pp. 67, 92–4. For further discussion of the rise of planning, management and scientific methodologies see also Becky Conekin, Frank Mort and Chris Waters, *Moments of Modernity: Reconstructing Britain 1945–1964* (London: Rivers Oram Press, 1999); Rose, *Governing the Soul*; Clapson, *Suburbs.*
6 Hilda Brown, 'Some Effects of Shift Work on Social and Domestic Life', *Yorkshire Bulletin of Economic and Social Research*, Occasional paper No. 2 (1959): preface, p. 2.
7 Samantha Lay, *British Social Realism: From Documentary to Brit-Grit* (London: New York: Wallflower, 2002), p. 11. Arthur Marwick, 'The

1960s: Was There a "Cultural Revolution"?', *Contemporary Record* 2, 3 (1988): p. 19, https://doi.org/10.1080/13619468808580986.

8 Penny Summerfield, 'Divisions at Sea: Class, Gender, Race, and Nation in Maritime Films of the Second World War, 1939–60', *Twentieth Century British History* (2011), p. 10, https://doi.org/10.1093/tcbh/hwr001; Philip Gillett, *The British Working Class in Postwar Film* (Manchester: Manchester University Press, 2003), p. 2.

9 Jeffrey Richard, 'New Waves and Old Myths: British Cinema in the 1960s', in Bart Moore-Gilbert and John Seed (eds) *Cultural Revolution? The Challenge of the Arts in the 1960s* (London: Routledge, 1992), p. 172.

10 Haggett, *Desperate Housewives*, p. 85.

11 D5284, 'Diary for 6 November' (1941), MOA, University of Sussex.

12 D5284, 'Diary for 7 November' (1941), MOA, University of Sussex.

13 D5284, 'Diary for 8 December' (1944), MOA, University of Sussex.

14 Elizabeth Wilson, *Only Half-Way to Paradise: Women in Postwar Britain, 1945–1968* (London: Tavistock, 1980), p. 50.

15 Alison Blunt and Robyn Dowling, *Home* (Hoboken: Taylor and Francis, 2012), p. 10; Shelley Mallett, 'Understanding Home: A Critical Review of the Literature', *The Sociological Review* 52, 1 (2004): pp. 68–9, https://doi.org/10.1111/j.1467-954X.2004.00442.x.

16 FR 2059, Will the Factory Girls Want to Stay Put or Go Home?, March 1944, MOA, University of Sussex, p. 6.

17 *Ibid.*, p. 3.

18 Gail Braybon and Penny Summerfield, *Out of the Cage: Women's Experiences in Two World Wars* (London: Pandora, 1987), p. 281.

19 D5284, 'Diary for 10 November' (1944), MOA, University of Sussex.

20 MOA FR 2059, Factory Girls, p. 5.

21 Haggett, *Desperate Housewives*, p. 89.

22 Vernon, 'Confidential Letter'. Penny Summerfield, 'Approaches to Women and Social Change in the Second World War', in Brian Brivati and Helen Jones (eds) *What Difference Did the War Make?* (London: Leicester University Press, 1993), p. 65.

23 Judy Giles, 'Narratives of Gender, Class, and Modernity in Women's Memories of Mid Twentieth Century Britain', *Signs* 28, 1 (2002): p. 22, https://doi.org/10.1086/340907. Judy Giles, 'Help for Housewives: Domestic Service and the Reconstruction of Domesticity in Britain, 1940–50', *Women's History Review* 10, 2 (1 June 2001): p. 29, https://doi.org/10.1080/09612020100200282. Stacey Gillis and Joanne Hollows, *Feminism, Domesticity and Popular Culture* (New York; London: Routledge, 2009), pp. 4–6.

24 Brown, 'Shift Work', preface.
25 *Ibid.*, p. 25.
26 *Ibid.*, pp. 25, 37.
27 *Ibid.*, p. 26.
28 Ministry of Labour and National Service, 'Report of Committee on Double Day-Shift Working' (Cmd 7147, June 1947), pp. 8–12.
29 Brown, 'Shift Work', pp. 8, 11.
30 Helen McCarthy, 'Social Science and Married Women's Employment in Post-War Britain', *Past & Present* 233, 1 (1 November 2016): p. 278, https://doi.org/10.1093/pastj/gtw035.
31 Judith Hubback, *Wives Who Went to College* (London: William Heinemann, 1957), p. 58.
32 Jackson, *Age of Stress*, p. 229.
33 Hubback, *Wives*, p. 67.
34 FR 1616, Some Psychological Factors in Home-Building, March 1943, MOA, University of Sussex, p. 12.
35 'Replies to March–April Directive Housework' (1951), MOA, University of Sussex, B4014.
36 MOA 'Housework', B016.
37 MOA 'Housework', F896.
38 Giles, 'Housewives', p. 301.
39 Violet Markham and Florence May Hancock, *Report on Post-War Organisation of Private Domestic Employment* (Ministry of Labour and National Service: HMSO, 1944), p. 7.
40 Violet Markham, 'Help for Housewives', *The Listener*, no. 900 (11 April 1946), p. 464.
41 Giles, 'Housewives', pp. 315–16.
42 Haggett, *Desperate Housewives*, p. 126.
43 Margaret Hughes, 'Letters to the Editor', *Manchester Guardian* (2 October 1954), p. 4.
44 Hughes, p. 4. Self-disciplined, 'Letters to the Editor', *Manchester Guardian* (11 October 1954), p. 4.
45 Joan Wise, 'Letters to the Editor', *Manchester Guardian* (5 October 1954), p. 6. Ash, *Nerves and the Nervous*, p. 191. Powell, *Sound Nerves*, p. 41.
46 Daisy Saunders, 'Letters to the Editor', *Manchester Guardian* (12 October 1954), p. 4.
47 Charlotte L. Loewenthal, 'Letters to the Editor', *Manchester Guardian* (6 October 1954), p. 6.
48 Jane Lewis, *The End of Marriage? Individualism and Intimate Relations* (Cheltenham; Northampton, MA: Edward Elgar, 2001), p. 85.

49 D5284, 'Diary for 5 November' (1944), MOA, University of Sussex.

50 Langhamer, *English in Love*, p. 181.

51 Janet Finch and Penny Summerfield, 'Social Reconstruction and the Emergence of Companionate Marriage, 1945–59', in David Clark (ed.) *Marriage, Domestic Life and Social Change: Writings for Jacqueline Burgoyne, 1944–88* (London: Routledge, 1991), p. 17.

52 Hughes, 'Letters to the Editor'.

53 Clapson, *Suburbs*, p. 49.

54 *Ibid.*, p. 45.

55 'Suburban Neurosis Up to Date', *The Lancet* 1, 18 January (1958): p. 146, http://dx.doi.org/10.1016/S0140-6736(58)90739-6.

56 Sidney P. W. Chave, 'Mental Health in Harlow New Town', *Journal of Psychosomatic Research* 10, 1 (1966): p. 39, https://doi.org/10.1016/0022-3999(66)90134-6.

57 Michael Dunlop Young and Peter Willmott, *Family and Kinship in East London* (London: Routledge & Kegan Paul, 1957); Mark Clapson, *Suburban Century: Social Change and Urban Growth in England and the United States* (Oxford: Berg, 2003), p. 127.

58 Chave, 'Mental Health', p. 43.

59 Klickmann, *Mending Your Nerves*, pp. 129–30.

60 Chave, 'Mental Health', p. 43.

61 Ineichen, 'Neurotic Wives', p. 481.

62 *Ibid.*, p. 485.

63 Hayward, 'Desperate Housewives', p. 55.

64 Klickmann, *Mending Your Nerves*, p. 37.

65 *Ibid.*, pp. 50, 126.

66 Henry Baruch Harris, *How to Live With Your Nerves and Like It: A Family Doctor Book* (London: British Medical Association, 1956), p. 19.

67 FR 2285, Women's Reasons for Having Small Families, September 1945, MOA, University of Sussex, p. 10.

68 Hannah Gavron, *The Captive Wife: Conflicts of Housebound Mothers* (London: Routledge & Kegan Paul, 1966).

69 *Ibid.*, p. 105.

70 *Ibid.*, p. 81.

71 *Ibid.*, p. 51.

72 *Ibid.*, p. 56.

73 FR 3110, General Attitudes to Sex, April 1949, MOA, University of Sussex, p. 10.

74 Claire Langhamer, *Women's Leisure in England, 1920–60* (Manchester: Manchester University Press, 2000), p. 133.

75 Allport, *Demobbed*, p. 3.

76 MOA FR 2285, Small Families, p. 6.

77 FR 2495, The State of Matrimony, June 1947, MOA, University of Sussex, p. 15.

78 P. G. Gray, 'The Housing Waiting Lists (England and Wales): An Inquiry Carried Out in July 1949 for the Ministry of Health' (Ministry of Health, 1949), The National Archives.

79 MOA FR 2495, Matrimony, p. 16.

80 Gray, 'Waiting Lists', p. 19.

81 Rachel M. Pierce, 'Marriage in the Fifties', *The Sociological Review* 11, 2 (1963): p. 233, https://doi.org/10.1111/j.1467-954X.1963.tb01232.x.

82 *Ibid.*, p. 238.

83 *Ibid.*, p. 236.

84 Paul Johnson, 'Introduction: Britain, 1900–1990', in Paul Johnson (ed.) *Twentieth-Century Britain: Economic, Social and Cultural Change* (London; New York: Longman, 1997), p. 11.

85 'The Rare Bird', *Daily Mirror* (7 May 1962), p. 21.

86 'Drama for the Millions', *Observer* (22 April 1962), p. 22.

87 *Ibid.*; 'The Rare Bird', p. 21.

88 Lynn Spigel, 'The Domestic Economy of Television Viewing in Postwar America', *Critical Studies in Mass Communication* 6, 4 (1989): p. 340, https://doi.org/10.1080/15295038909366761. Although specifically working with US sources, Spigel's broad arguments about the contradictory responses to the reception of television in the home appear relevant to the UK context.

89 Ted Kotcheff, 'Where I Live' (ABC for ITV, 1960).

90 Elizabeth Roberts, *Women and Families: An Oral History, 1940–1970* (Oxford: Blackwell, 1995), p. 19. Roberts argues that the proportion of elderly in the community increased in the post-Second World War period with a concomitant effect on women's caring responsibilities.

91 John Hill, 'From the "New Wave" to "Brit-Grit": Continuity and Difference in Working-Class Realism', in Justine Ashby and Andrew Higson (eds) *British Cinema: Past and Present* (London: Routledge, 2000), p. 250; John Schlesinger, *A Kind of Loving* (Vic Films Productions, 1962); Karel Reisz, *Saturday Night and Sunday Morning* (Woodfall Film Productions, 1960); Tony Richardson, *The Loneliness of the Long Distance Runner* (Woodfall Film Productions, 1962).

92 'A Winner All the Way', *Daily Mirror* (13 April 1962), p. 21. *Saturday Night and Sunday Morning* won a BAFTA for best British film in 1961 and *A Kind of Loving* was nominated for four BAFTAs in 1964, including best film. 'British Academy of Film and Television Arts Awards Database',

19 April 2016, http://awards.bafta.org/. Accessed 17 May 2017. *A Kind of Loving* also won the Golden Bear at the Berlin Film Festival.

93 Melanie Bell, *Femininity in the Frame: Women and 1950s British Popular Cinema* (London: IBTauris, 2010), p. 11.

94 Stephen C. Shafer, 'An Overview of the Working Classes in British Feature Film from the 1960s to the 1980s: From Class Consciousness to Marginalization', *International Labor and Working-Class History*, 59 (2001): p. 7, https://doi.org/10.2307/27672706.

95 *Ibid.*, p. 8. Arthur Marwick, 'Room at the Top, Saturday Night and Sunday Morning, and the "Cultural Revolution" in Britain', *Journal of Contemporary History* 19, 1 (1984): pp. 148–9, https://doi.org/10.117 7/002200948401900107.

96 *Ibid.*, p. 130.

97 Danny Powell, *Studying British Cinema: The 1960s* (Leighton Buzzard: Auteur Publishing, 2009), p. 56.

98 'All Our Own Work', *The Times* (28 April 1962), p. 9.

99 '"X" Film Show at Commons', *Daily Mirror* (30 May 1962), p. 21.

100 Bell, *Femininity*, 11; Richard, 'New Waves', p. 172.

101 Summerfield, 'Divisions at Sea', p. 10; Gillett, *British Working Class*, p. 2.

102 Shafer, 'Working Classes in British Feature Film', p. 6; Bill Osgerby, *Youth in Britain since 1945* (Oxford: Blackwell, 1998), p. 33.

103 Selina Todd and Hilary Young, 'Baby-Boomers to "Beanstalkers"', *Cultural & Social History* 9, 3 (2012): p. 452, https://doi.org/10.2752/147800412X13347542916747. Gillian A. M. Mitchell, 'Reassessing "the Generation Gap": Bill Hayley's 1957 Tour of Britain, Inter-Generational Relations and Attitudes to Rock 'n' Roll in the Late 1950s', *Twentieth Century British History* (2013), pp. 16–17, https://doi.org/10.1093/tcbh/hwt013.

104 Bell, *Femininity*, p. 69.

105 'New Author and Old Outlook: The First Notable Alignment', *Guardian* (14 May 1962), p. 16.

106 Stuart Laing, *Representations of Working-Class Life 1957–1964* (Basingstoke: Macmillan, 1986), p. 131.

107 Karel Reisz, *Saturday Night and Sunday Morning*.

108 Tony Richardson, *The Loneliness of the Long Distance Runner*.

109 Spigel, 'Television Viewing', p. 340.

110 1,182 million cinema audience in 1955 versus 501 million in 1960 and a growth from 4,503 TV licence holders to 10,469 in the same period. Patricia Perilli, 'Statistical Survey of the British Film Industry', in James

Curran and Vincent Porter (eds) *British Cinema History* (London: Weidenfeld and Nicholson, 1983), p. 372.

111 Marwick, 'Room at the Top', p. 147; Gray, 'Waiting Lists'.
112 *People's Homes*, p. 198.
113 John Hill, 'Working Class Realism and Sexual Reaction: Some Theses on the British "New Wave"', in Curran and Porter (eds) *British Cinema History*, p. 305.
114 James Chapman, 'Our Finest Hour Revisited: The Second World War in British Feature Films since 1945', *Journal of Popular British Cinema* 1 (1998): p. 67. Quoted in Summerfield, 'Divisions at Sea', p. 2.
115 D5284, 'Letter to MO 1942'.

5

The democratisation of stress: popular and personal discourse in the 1960s and 1970s

> I knew when I got to Birmingham that I was up against some cracking students in ability and I knew I would have to work me socks off and I did, but unfortunately I found it got to me, and I suspect it was the first sign in me life of nervous tension. It did get to me, and I can remember in my last year I had to go to the doctors once or twice. I didn't realise it at the time but I wasn't sleeping particularly well but it was all, I realise now it was all evidence of stress.[1]

This was Jeff Mills's description of his experience as a student at Birmingham University in the late 1950s given as part of a life history interview in 1998. Born in 1938, Jeff was the son of a miner from Westhoughton in Lancashire and one of the 2.6 per cent of eighteen-year-olds from working-class homes who went to university in the period.[2] By the late 1950s, the number of students attending university in Britain had almost doubled compared to before the war, but students from working-class homes were still very much in a minority. With no family experience of higher education, Jeff perceived university life as extremely competitive, struggled socially and had high expectations of what he should be achieving. As he explained, 'I don't think me parents, then, understood the system, or, I'm not decrying them, I mean I was on my own you see.'[3] Underpinning Jeff's time at Birmingham was an anxiety that the experience had to be worth the time, effort and sacrifice that had got him there.

Although he did not realise it, Jeff was not alone in experiencing 'nervous tension' as a student. The *Daily Mirror* reported its alarm in 1953 that 'worry' was affecting 'as many as one in five younger people' and that much of this was due to 'Stress, that modern illness caused by working too long at top pressure.'[4] Ten years later the same newspaper reported from a BMA conference in Oxford that 'An early warning system is needed to detect excessive mental strain in Britain's most brilliant university students.' According to Dr Ronald Still, responsible for the health of students at Leeds University, 'Once I had the naïve idea that hard work did nobody any harm. I no longer take this view, I think hard mental work does sometimes cause mental disturbance.'[5] While such an idea was partly a re-emergence of the old neurasthenic connection between 'brain work' and nervous suffering what was new was its application to this more demographically diverse population of students, benefiting from the educational reforms of post-war Britain. Also novel was the very openness of the discussion about mental health in one of Britain's most widely read newspapers.[6]

Jeff's experience and the concerns being raised about the student population of the 1950s and 1960s illustrate the ways in which the concept of stress was becoming much more common within popular discourse and how ideas about stress were initially focused on certain sections of the population, revealing a continuity with much earlier ideas about status and nervous disorders. By examining newspaper coverage of stress between the 1950s and 1970s, this chapter shows how ideas about the causes and sufferers of stress became a visible part of popular culture and an explanation for certain types of negative experience. Analysis of personal testimony from contemporary sufferers then illustrates the time lag between stress as part of public discourse and its adoption by individuals to describe their own experiences.

Newspaper reporting

Newspapers offer a particularly useful way of understanding the growing presence of stress in popular culture because until the 1970s they were at the heart of that culture. With most adults reading at least one national paper, such newspapers had a social and cultural authority that enabled them to reflect and shape attitudes and contribute to the social, economic and cultural shifts in late twentieth-century Britain that were the context for the increase in stress.[7] However, while at the mid-century Britons read more newspapers per capita than any other people in the world, the history of newspapers in Britain in the second half of the twentieth century was also one of decline.[8] In order to maintain their popularity in the post-war period, particularly as television became more and more important, newspapers increasingly sought to connect with the everyday experiences of their audiences by opening up discussion of topics previously considered private.[9] This was evident in the growing coverage of health and, more often, ill-health-related topics, including stress. Stress was offered as an explanation for the variety of responses that people had to everyday life experiences: an explanation that effectively problematised areas of working and domestic life, previously accepted as normal, and often private. This reframing of problematic experiences as stress helped to both popularise the concept and increase the number of sufferers, the availability of a new, medical label tending to encourage adoption.[10]

From the 1960s onwards, newspaper coverage of stress in tabloid and broadsheet national newspapers initially emphasised the high status of those prone to stress, in keeping with older discourses around neurasthenia. However, this was very soon expanded to suggest that anyone from any walk of life was susceptible to stress. This both fuelled and reflected the growing popular understanding of everyday stress, providing a framework and language which enabled individuals to negotiate new interpretations of their own troublesome experiences. Arguably newspapers and magazines in the UK lagged behind US publications, which, according to Watkins, were already highlighting the problem of stress in periodicals such as *Reader's Digest*, *Newsweek* and even *Vogue* in the 1950s, reflecting the growing research activity in science, industry and the military in the USA.[11] As the last chapter showed, many everyday life experiences were increasingly being problematised or understood in medicalised ways. At the same time there was increased interest in health and ill-health stories in newspapers and coverage of previously taboo issues such as mental health, all of which created the context for a sense that life was becoming more mentally challenging.

As the discussion about students at the beginning of this chapter highlighted, stress was initially framed by newspaper reports as a disease of particular elite groups. Indeed, many of the hard-working students of such concern to Dr Still at the Oxford conference in 1963 may well have gone on to form the nucleus of another group, identified in newspaper reports as particularly at risk from the pressures of their work; the businessman or business executive. Almost always male, white and middle-class, an article in 1960 referred to the popular belief that 'the boss got more "stress disorders" than those working under him', although it did admit that the evidence for this was incomplete.[12] Similarly, 'the ageing worker and executive' featured in the 1963 edition of *Human Relations in Modern Industry* by Dr Tredgold of Roffey Park as a category of employee particularly susceptible to mental deterioration and less able to adapt to the pressure of life and rapid change.[13] Perhaps responding to similar concerns, in 1960 the *Guardian* reported the creation of an executive retreat at Ruthin Castle in Wales modelled on similar American institutions, and aimed at important businessmen working under pressure. Such facilities had been available in the USA for some time, with an advertisement in the *New York Times* in the early 1940s offering businessmen whose success had led to high tension and 'jangled nerves' a stay at a resort in Hot Springs, Virginia.[14] Indeed, the idea of a rest cure was common to many early twentieth-century self-help books, but what was different here was the specific connection between high-status businessmen, their success and stress. Ruthin Castle offered a week's stay under medical supervision, with a medical check-up, rest and relaxation in a country-house atmosphere at fifty-five guineas for a private luxury room. At that price, this was obviously only available to the wealthy or those whose organisations were paying. As the vice-chairman of the Board of Governors of Ruthin Castle Centre Ltd explained to the *Guardian*, a man 'of the beer and public house type, a man of no culture whatsoever, would hardly fit in', reinforcing the sense of exclusivity but also underpinning the connection between status and stress.[15] Ruthin Castle was apparently a more upmarket, though rather less democratic version of the Rehabilitation Centre at Roffey Park. The article concluded that 'it may well be that a visit to Ruthin will become an accepted part of the senior British executive's life, a status symbol in an age when stress is the affliction of successful indispensables'.[16] This privileging of the mental suffering of the social and business elite clearly discounted any possibility that those in less elevated positions might also suffer stress and is illustrative of the continuing hold of Britain's class structure on ideas about work and health.

That such a centre was needed was suggested by a 1968 Institute of Director's (IoD) survey, reported in the *Daily Mirror*, which had shown '250 out of 2,000 directors were judged to be under stress', attributing this not just to work, but to the inadequacies of their wives'

support for them.[17] This latter point apparently arose from the fact
that many directors were self-made men who had married young and
whose business success had led to an increased social status that their
wives were ill-equipped to navigate successfully. Thus 'the stress of
situations at home led to twice as much anxiety among the directors
as stress at work'.[18] Notably, no comment was made regarding the
effect of such stress on their wives, whose experience was deemed less
important as they were not running large institutions or contributing
to the national economy. Another *Daily Mirror* article reported that
doctors and psychiatrists were worried by the growing impact of 'stress
and tension in this age of anxiety', and attributed 'mental and emotional
crack-ups' to both the fear of nuclear annihilation and 'the effort to
keep up with the Joneses'.[19] Fear of nuclear war was very real and
harnessed in public discourse both by those who wished to build up
Britain's nuclear arsenal and by those who opposed it. It permeated
into popular culture and, as Bourke has argued, was part of more
general fears about the military, scientists and computing, all of which
contributed to a stressful modern environment.[20] Concern about
'keeping up with the Joneses' echoed some of the earlier concerns
raised about suburban neurosis and women being over-house-proud
and highlights contemporary unease about consumerism and social
mobility. As discussed in the last chapter, women in the post-war period
were experiencing their own stress at home, sometimes, but not always,
fuelled by the actions or inactions of husbands and the IoD's findings
would seem to confirm a picture of the complex interplay between
women's domestic work, male employment and the effects of changing
class identities.

There was a sense too in newspaper reporting that the world had
fundamentally changed and that this too was perhaps contributing to a
mounting sense that modern life was stressful. *The Daily Mirror* reported
on a new National Marriage Guidance Council booklet targeting the
problems facing middle-aged couples, explaining that 'For the majority
life has changed considerably in the past 40 or 50 years and for some,
modern conditions bring a mental stress harder to cope with than
physical illness.'[21] This assertion that 'modern conditions' were somehow
more stressful was yet another repetition of the concerns raised by
Ash much earlier in the century.[22] The idea that people in each decade
were seeing more change, happening more rapidly and suffering as a

result, would be repeated frequently throughout the century, appearing often in personal accounts of stress at its end. Declaring life to be more stressful was effectively a comment on the speed of change and the sense of powerlessness of the individual in the face of such change. For the self-help authors of the early twentieth century, there had been a growing disquiet amongst the professional middle class about the rapidity of change and its social impact. Economic and technological change had brought opportunity and new possibilities for the ambitious that some perceived as a threat to the social order. Similarly, 1960s Britain with its high employment levels and socially mobile post-war generation was also changing and it was often easier to explain people's disquiet about such change by pathologising their response rather than addressing the underlying causes of their discomfort.

The subject of stress appeared to provide useful copy for newspapers, expanding beyond the troubles of high-powered business executives and their wives, and reflecting developments in stress research that now focused on assessing personality types and measuring stressful life events and their impact on health.[23] Indeed, a 1972 article in the *Daily Mirror* outlined the 'seven ages of stress', explaining that 'the increasing pressures of life have created the second fastest-growing disease of the twentieth century: mental stress'. Linked to a National Association for Mental Health campaign, the article identified seven ages from toddler to old age and argued that at every life stage the individual could fall foul of life experiences that could trigger not just stress, but other mental illnesses too.[24] This shift of emphasis now implied that there was no age when the threat of stress was not present, but more significantly stress was now being positioned as something that anyone might experience, not just the executive or 'successful indispensables', who visited Ruthin Castle.[25] 'Stress has become the dirty word of the Seventies. Everyone suffers from it', declared another feature on the women's page of the *Daily Mirror*, illustrated by a photograph of a woman apparently tearing her hair out. The article went on to explain, 'This deadly six letter word is as much a part of your day as breathing', but offered limited ideas for dealing with stress, including spending more time with family and trying to change a boring job.[26]

By 1976, under a headline of 'Stress: the big danger to your health', the *Daily Mirror* identified how a whole family might be stressed: 'Dad has an unrewarding job on a production line, Mum's trapped in a tower block flat with thin walls. Their son is on the dole. The daughter is doing exams. Gran still can't cope with the new money. And they live next to a motorway.'[27] Now it was not just the pressure of high-level business decisions that might cause stress, but the tedium of a pro-duction-line job, the inconveniences of tower-block living, the hopeless-ness of unemployment, anxiety of examinations and the challenges of decimalisation and a noisy environment: seven ages of stress indeed. The same article did not abandon the figure of the stressed executive, but instead, while acknowledging stress as 'an occupational hazard for overworked business executives weighed down with the burden of responsibility', it suggested that they were 'far better able to cope with stress than an ordinary working-class person'.[28] Thus status dif-ference was maintained: the executive was better able to manage stress, presumably because he had the potential of a trip to somewhere like Ruthin Castle, which 'Dad' certainly did not, and also because he had more than ten years of journalists telling him his work was making him ill, whereas the working man's job had apparently only just become stressful. Such shifts in emphasis reflected the blurring of class boundaries, an increasing emphasis on health and safety and greater union focus on psychological as well as physical health. By 1988, a trade union-funded research report was quoted in the *Guardian* claiming to 'explode the myth of stress as an executive disease', explaining that 'Illnesses caused by stress are more likely to strike manual and clerical workers, particularly women, than the hard-pressed businessman as had generally been supposed.'[29] Somewhat late to the party and appar-ently casting aside previous suspicions about organisational welfare mentioned in Chapter 3, the unions perhaps perceived the potential of stress as leverage in their increasingly difficult dealings with 1980s management.

Fears about loss of employment identified yet another susceptible group, as a *Daily Mirror* report commented in 1980: 'family doctors in areas where unemployment is hitting hardest are beginning to see more patients with stress symptoms brought about by worry over losing a job'.[30] If such worries came true then being unemployed also created susceptibility to stress, as the same article entitled, 'Death on the dole … the new threat' announced new research into 'the impact of a wide range of stresses on the unemployed'.[31] How helpful or otherwise it was to the already worried unemployed to be told they now risked the new problem of stress is debatable. It is evident from personal testimony that the unemployed themselves did connect their lack of work to mental health issues, as two responses to MOP directives in the early 1980s illustrate. A civil servant who had worked for thirty years before losing his job wrote, 'I celebrated redundancy by going into a slow nervous breakdown culminating in [an] unsuccessful suicide attempt.'[32] The second, a fifty-nine-year-old ex-banker, told MOP, 'In January 1979 I suffered a nervous breakdown as a result of work pressures and travelling conditions and was retired by my employers in May of that year as a direct result of my GP's recommendation.' He went on to explain that the process of registering as unemployed and going through a number of unsuccessful redeployment interviews with the then Manpower Commission was 'just as pressure making' and so he chose not to sign on to the unemployment register after 1979, but to get by on an early pension.[33] It is notable that while both respondents talked about the effects of unemployment, neither used the word 'stress' despite its prevalence in contemporary culture.

Many of the newspaper stories that featured stress were gleaned from medical and academic research where stress had become critical to understanding the effects of social conditions on mental and physical health in the post-war era.[34] They also reflected the way in which popular psychology increasingly focused on individual lifestyles.[35] Newspapers were bringing the language of stress into the mainstream, so it is not surprising that their deployment of the concept and language was ahead of the layperson's. Before the 1960s, stress usually referred to an external cause of discomfort; for example, a *Daily Mirror* article in 1940 written by the paper's psychologist about the effects of fear talked about people's reactions to 'anxiety and stress and danger'.[36] It explained the functioning of adrenalin in dangerous situations and was evidently intended to calm a readership suffering the strategic bombing of Britain. Stress as a medical condition and as a description of both cause and resulting experience only came into usage following Selye's work in the 1950s.[37] In popular culture, the language of nerves continued to dominate in the 1960s and 1970s. Contemporary self-help books talked about nerves; for example, the extremely successful *Self-help for Your Nerves* by Australian GP Dr Claire Weekes, published in 1962 and reprinted multiple times in the following decades, referred to 'nervous breakdown' and nerves being 'in a bad way', rarely mentioning stress at all.[38] Weekes was the author of dozens of self-help books focusing on nervous conditions, many continuing in print well into the twenty-first century. Her books and audio recordings avoided medical language in favour of terms such as 'nerves' and 'nervous illness' even when stress had become the ubiquitous catch-all term for many of the conditions she addressed.[39]

Similarly, published in the late 1960s, *Do Something about Those Nerves* by Dr R. A. B. Rorie, a British family doctor, referred throughout the book to 'nerves' in quotation marks and only used the word stress to refer to the external causes of 'breakdown'.[40] As discussed in Chapter 1, the emphasis in many such books was on writing for a lay reader, and Rorie's book emphasised its 'simple straightforward language'.[41] Thus, such books reflected the terminology that people used every day to explain their feelings and experiences, which was largely still the helpfully vague lexicon of nerves, using 'nervous breakdown', 'nervous conditions' and 'nerves' to describe a variety of experiences, as Jeff Mill's talk of 'nervous tension' showed at the beginning of the chapter. Newspaper reporting reflected the evolution from nerves to stress, often drawing on both the medical and social scientific terminology together with the lay language of ordinary people in the same articles. It is notable that terms revolving around nerves and stress were both used to describe the same types of situations and symptoms, and both had the same mutability in labelling a wide range of experiences. The difference was that stress was the more contemporary term and carried with it the validity of current medical and psychological use.

Prescription drugs

Running parallel with the public discussion about stress was a critical view of the increasing use of prescription drugs to tackle the problem. A series of *Daily Mirror* articles in the mid-1950s, written in a somewhat sensationalist tone and focusing on GPs prescribing sleeping pills, had asked, 'Are they wrong in helping their patients to bear the stress of life more easily?' and quoted a busy city centre chemist claiming, 'Only today I have sent out 400 tablets – THREE QUARTERS OF THEM FOR SOOTHING FRAYED NERVES.'[42] The companion piece the following day explained that 'The drug-takers are victims of a disease peculiar to civilisation called STRESS' and explained the 'flight or fight' theory. While it went on to clarify the different uses of barbiturates and amphetamines for dealing with such problems, it bemoaned the fact that such drugs were the result of poor psychiatric provision within the NHS: 'Only about five or six teaching hospitals take psychiatric patients – and they have waiting lists of from three to six months. For the rest, the only way to get treatment from a psychiatrist is to be an out-patient at a mental hospital. And few people relish that idea.'[43] Certainly, the continuing stigma around mental health issues meant that for many people a prescription for drugs was far more acceptable than engaging with NHS psychiatric services, and little occurred to change that between the 1950s and 1970s.

A 1970 article in *Science* magazine claimed that the pharmaceutical industry was deliberately redefining and relabelling a range of human behaviours that until recently had been seen as the normal ups and downs of human existence, as medical problems to be treated with drugs.[44] According to a contemporary report in one medical journal, the annual prescribing of Valium in Britain had increased by 4.1 million prescriptions during the period 1965 to 1970, while prescriptions for other minor and major tranquillisers showed an increase of 25 per cent, with the overall increase in tranquilliser prescribing reaching 59 per cent.[45] As the authors of the journal article themselves commented, the usefulness of such drugs was controversial because of the problems in defining what patients were actually suffering from and whether the treatment addressed it. They also suggested that the increase in prescribing was influenced by more than just the number of patients presenting with conditions that were treatable with tranquillisers. Their survey of GPs revealed twice as many women being prescribed psychotropic drugs than men and they suggested further that more focused research was needed to understand this prescribing pattern.[46] While some of the increase in prescriptions could be attributed to the frequency and duration of treatment, the fact that such drugs were marketed as addressing a wide range of conditions also contributed to their popularity.[47] Arguably this was also linked to the pharmaceutical companies' need to bring new drugs to market as patents ran out and generic formulations of their previously star products became available. Thus, they heavily promoted new drugs, which meant the replacement of old drugs by new ones which, according to Shorter, were often less efficacious.[48] Additionally, Healy has suggested that pharmaceutical companies also began effectively to market diseases rather than their treatments and that this contributed both to the medicalisation of trivial complaints and the increase in prescription drug use.[49]

By the mid-1980s, *The Times* was pursuing the argument that pharmaceutical companies were benefiting, suggesting that 'Stress and anxiety seem to be the plague of modern society. The pharmaceutical industry has certainly found it to be one of the most profitable illnesses.' The article went on to criticise the extensive use of Valium and other tranquillisers to deal with stress, hinting that this was one of the factors behind the apparent explosion in psychological problems.[50] Certainly if there appeared to be effective treatments for people's suffering, it might seem reasonable that they would be more likely to ask their GP for such treatment. Ironically, it was around this time that concerns were starting to be aired in newspapers about the risks of dependency in Valium use which, according to Healy, contributed to the rapid decline in use of benzodiazepines (the category to which Valium belongs) and the rise of less effective anti-depressants.[51] Arguably, it was the confluence of increasing consumerism, sophisticated advertising and marketing techniques, as well as media reporting that was contributing to the sense that what had been part of the inevitable troubles of life was now something that needed addressing, and in many cases, addressing with prescription drugs.

Feeling the strain

Personal accounts of stress such as Jeff Mill's highlighted at the beginning of this chapter, and related in life history interviews, reveal that although the popular and public discourse of stress increased during this period, there was a delay between the appearance and use of such terminology and concepts in the media, and individuals applying such notions to themselves. Individual testimonies taken from collections of oral history interviews recorded in the late 1990s provide accounts of the symptoms of stress, perceived causes and the responses of colleagues, friends and the stressed themselves to what they were experiencing. As Haggett has pointed out, it has traditionally been assumed that women are 'more naturally predisposed' to depression and anxiety disorders, and hence men's experience and coping strategies are less well understood. These accounts are all by men and all relate their stress to their work and offer insight into the relatively obscure world of how men have experienced and coped with personal and professional pressures. They provide insight into the ways in which men's experiences of mental health problems were often hidden behind somatic symptoms and suggest concerns about the threat that such problems posed to conceptions of masculine identity.[52]

These accounts also reveal how the responses of others were important in the acknowledgement or denial of an individual's stress and that the locations where stress appeared were often those which were more socially or culturally acceptable, as seen in the cases of Robert W and Margaret S at Roffey Park in the 1940s in Chapter 3. Reactions to those who were stressed varied from sympathetic to suspicious and highlight how slowly values were changing. The generations who lived through the Second World War and brought up children in its aftermath continued to adhere to a norm of stoicism and privacy that was wary of the psychological and emotional, however much popular culture seemed to embrace them. While the public discourse of stress was becoming more and more common, the private understanding of the concept and its application to everyday life were still limited. Personal accounts also illustrate lay use of terminology, stress being retrospectively applied to experiences, which as these stories reveal, were more often explained in terms of nerves and breakdown at the time. As such they support the idea that the 1970s was a transitional decade during which the public discourse of stress increased, but the adoption of the term and concept had not yet become common in everyday life.

The first account comes from Ken Duckworth who came to Britain from Sri Lanka in the late 1950s and joined the Civil Service, where he soon progressed from a clerical role to Executive Officer. Ken began to struggle with his duties and his boss at the time was concerned enough to suggest demotion to relieve Ken of some of the pressure of work, which he gladly accepted. For a time, he was well; however, he eventually accepted a promotion again and very soon found that the new role was 'causing me a great deal of stress being a manager of people'. As Ken explained, 'I kept going and thinking, "Oh God I'm not doing well in my job." My people who worked under [me] were not doing right as well. They were making mistakes, I was trying to correct their mistakes and the work started piling up on me and I started taking sick leave, too much stress.'[53] He approached his new manager who told him to 'stop moaning, try and do my job and stop worrying'. Unsurprisingly, this did not resolve matters and Ken reported having 'dreadful feeling, didn't want to go to work, scared, scared that I might have a bad day. Feeling worried, how I could manage my staff, how I could make them happy, and make them do their work well and me be in charge of them.' Eventually, this came to a head and 'one day I just cracked up'. He ended up under medical supervision and 'taking lots of Valium ... they don't give Valium so much now, but I was on Valium and some other stuff'.[54]

Ultimately, Ken's story took a turn for the worse and he went on to suffer from serious mental health problems and to spend time in various institutions. However, his account of his experience of stress in the 1960s illustrates several of the issues arising in the contemporary media coverage and popular understanding. First, the use of Valium to deal with his stress would seem to fit with the pattern of increased prescribing reported by the media. Second, despite his job title of 'executive', Ken's was not a particularly senior role and he did not fulfil the stereotype of the high-powered business executive. Third, although his first boss appeared sympathetic and willing to accommodate Ken's struggles, by relieving him of some responsibilities, his new boss showed a lack of understanding and assumptions about stress as something that the individual could overcome through willpower: a view very similar to those expressed by Welfare Officer Miss Richmond in the 1940s, in Chapter 3. It is evident that Ken had little control over his situation, was not skilled at managing other people, which made his responsibilities more overwhelming, and was not viewed particularly sympathetically by his manager. His case is also consistent with later research carried out among civil servants by the London School of Hygiene and Tropical Medicine and referred to as the Whitehall studies. This work was intended to track social determinants of health and mortality rates and was carried out over a ten-year period from the late 1960s and then repeated in the 1980s. What became apparent from its results was that those with lower-status roles, who had low control over their own jobs, little opportunity to learn and develop skills and less variety at work, all had a higher risk of stress and cardiovascular disease.[55] Although Ken's case predated the studies, his experience of stress certainly fitted its findings.

For other stress sufferers, it was not just lack of control or understanding from a boss, but a sense that people were suspicious of claims of
stress that characterised responses and reinforced the privileging of
physical over psychological symptoms of ill-health. Peter Allen was in
his early twenties and working in his first supervisory role in charge
of sixty local authority gardeners in Hull. With little idea of how to
manage people, he copied the tough and authoritarian style of his
own boss, with damaging results. He explained what happened in
an interview in 1998 carried out as part of the Millennium Memory
Bank project, recording the lives of ordinary people from all over
Britain. 'I went off. I just collapsed one day, I just keeled over one day
and I went home, and I was taken home, and the doctor said: "Oh
you've had a nervous breakdown." I didn't know what it was, there
wasn't anything broken or twisted or anything, your lungs weren't
bad it was a nervous breakdown.'[56] Peter's account acknowledged
his physical symptoms (collapsing) but shows, more than twenty
years after the event, his continued puzzlement at the psychological
diagnosis he was given. His attempt to understand what was meant by
the rather vague term, 'nervous breakdown', focused on the absence
of physical impairment. His model of understanding illness was
predicated on visible physical symptoms, as was that of many of his
contemporaries, as he explained: 'In those days well people just used
to say "he's had a nervous breakdown" and for the first two hours
they were very sympathetic, but after that it was, you know, it's not
like a broken leg if you can't see it, if it's not manifest then people,
if it's in your head, can't quite understand it.' His account illustrates
the point that people were mistrustful of diagnoses without visible
symptoms, seeing claims to stress as excuses for an unacceptable
lack of stoicism or a form of malingering. It also reflects the fact
that despite the growing popular discourse of stress, it was poorly
understood or recognised among people going about their lives in the
early 1970s.

Elsewhere in Peter's interview his views expressed both continuity
and change regarding attitudes:

> I think this still happens today, unless you've been in those situations
> it's very hard to understand how, how people react to them, and I hear
> these days people say 'he's gone off with his', what do we call it now,
> we call it pressure, stress that's it, stress, 'gone off with stress', and

people say 'well I don't know why he's stressed, he don't do anything'.
You know that sort of thing. But people don't realise that stress is brought
on by a lot of different things.

Struggling to find the correct, contemporary term for his historical
experience, eventually identifying 'stress', it is evident that this was
not a term available or applied at the time of his experience in the
early 1970s. It seems that, in 1998, it was still new to Peter, and people's
responses to it persistently those of suspicion and dismissal.

Peter, like Ken, was also prescribed Valium by his doctor: 'I was
just put on long courses of Valium and things like that, tablets that
used to sort of wipe your mind out.' For him the experience was largely
negative, as he explained: 'when I did eventually go back to work it
was like I had to write everything down because any time you thought
of anything it was wiped off the blackboard, you see, this sort of thing,
so that took a lot of getting over did that'. Arguably, the side effects of
the medication were as pernicious as the condition they were supposed
to be treating, and certainly, Peter appeared to link his experience of
taking Valium with his lengthy recovery period. He explained that it
was 'very, very hard to go back to work, I was very frightened to go
back ... but I had one or two friends when I went back and they sort
of nursed me through the first period and then it got better and better,
but it scarred me for many years and I still fear certain situations that
I shouldn't'. It is hard to discount the additional fear that the mental
debility caused by Valium must have created for Peter, contributing
to the difficulty he felt in returning to work.

Looking back on his experience twenty-five years later, Peter
described it as 'quite a traumatic experience 'cos nobody really understood mental health very much', but he also framed it as 'part of your
learning curve and part of growing up'. His normalisation of his
experience as something to be learned reflected a stoicism about mental
suffering that was slow to change in the face of ongoing stigma about
mental ill-health. Nowhere in his account, did he reflect on the circumstances of the role he found himself in or the organisation's
responsibility to him, instead he effectively attributed his suffering to
a particular life-stage and his own inadequacy.[57]

At much the same time as Peter's breakdown, Jeff Mills, encountered
earlier in this chapter as a student at Birmingham University in the
1950s, was taking on a deputy headteacher role in Lancashire and

experiencing a range of symptoms that, despite previous events, he was slow to recognise as stress. At one point, driving home from work he had pains in his arms and chest and thought he was having a heart attack, opening his car door to ask a female passer-by for help, before thinking better of it and speeding home. Other symptoms included 'couldn't sleep, bad eyes, bad head. I kept going into work, I think I was doing my job, couldn't sleep at night but could sleep as soon as I came back from work.'[58] He was also having constant nightmares and eventually consulted his doctor who asked him about his marriage and financial situation, but who Jeff felt 'wasn't taking me seriously'. He was given 'some tablets' but these made his headaches worse, and he continued to work. Then as he explained,

> I suddenly discovered I wouldn't go into shops. I didn't want to go anywhere where there were people and yet I would go into school where there were lots of people. But I would not – we'd go to Bolton on a Saturday and I would sit in the car rather than go into a shop. Um, don't ask me what it was I just had feelings of terror, me mind would go blank, it was almost a fear I suppose.

Jeff's problem was that, like Peter, his framework for understanding his own health was a physical one, so he was focused on his physical symptoms and did not know what to make of more psychological ones, despite having had a similar experience as a student. Eventually, his father-in-law persuaded him to see a different doctor, who asked him about his symptoms and his job and, as Jeff reported, concluded, 'it's complete nervous exhaustion and stress, nothing but'. He prescribed different medication and signed Jeff off work for a fortnight.

While he needed to continue with medication, Jeff was able to return to work after this break, and summed up his experiences: 'I don't think the people at work ever knew. I don't think I ever showed it at work, I just coped, but out of work things were just falling apart.' It is notable that, according to him, Jeff's symptoms only appeared when he was not at work, despite his work being the cause of his stress. For him, there was perhaps just too much invested in his professional identity to allow symptoms to emerge during school hours. Instead, it was only when he was in a non-work context that they appeared. The reverse was the case, as discussed in Chapter 3, for one of the patients at Roffey Park who struggled with a difficult domestic situation that manifested itself as stress at work. What is evident is that the causes of stress and the places and times in which symptoms became manifest were not always directly connected. Indeed, stress often only became apparent away from its causes in circumstances that were less threatening to the sufferer's professional or personal identity or in which stress might be more easily validated. In Jeff's case it may also have been linked to his historical experiences of wishing to keep private his struggles and his own perception of shame at his inability to cope. It seems unlikely that no one at work noticed that Jeff was stressed, although, as he himself suggested, his own boss was 'going through, I think, a bit of stress himself' and was therefore perhaps less able to deal with the problems of a subordinate, especially one who was effectively filling in for his own shortcomings. Certainly, there was no institutional awareness or preparedness for such a contingency.

Indeed, Jeff himself did not really recognise the cause of his ills until afterwards when he acknowledged that 'what I didn't realise was that I was working too hard, I realise it now, but it's taken a long time. I was working so hard it was unbelievable.' Not unlike the views he expressed of himself as a student, he concluded that 'I was obviously trying to impress and I wanted to be a head and I was doing all sorts of courses.' Evidently, his ambition and desire to prove himself, this time to justify his promotion to deputy head and his desire for a head-ship, provided the basis for taking on too much work and becoming stressed. Like Peter, nowhere did Jeff question the organisational situation that enabled this to happen, nor the lack of support. Instead, his focus on his ability to continue working after his two weeks of sick leave was consistent with a sense of stoicism and persistence common to a generation who lived through the Second World War. Jeff alluded to a further experience of stress later in his career when he became a headmaster, but by then he could recognise his symptoms and was able to manage his stress: 'the one thing it taught me was that a) you mustn't take everything too seriously and b) you don't try and do everything yourself'. It seemed that as he got older, and achieved his ambitions, he was better able to understand his response to stressful situations, although he still saw everything in terms of managing himself and his own response, rather than addressing causative factors.[59]

All three accounts illustrate key elements of contemporary popular understanding (or lack of understanding) of stress in the 1960s and

1970s. They privileged physical symptoms over psychological ones, partly because they were easier to understand and interpret, but also because for many people the whole area of mental ill-health was one of stigma and taboo and best avoided for fear of any hint of madness. Aligned to this was a particular contemporary understanding of masculine identity as all three men were part of the post-war managerial generation who were expected to disavow any hint of being 'soft', which effectively meant living with the 'necessity to deny stress'.[60] This made it all the more difficult to deal with the very real fear that all three mentioned in their accounts, as men were not supposed to be prey to such emotions. Within such a prescriptive framework, it was difficult for them to acknowledge let alone be open about what they were experiencing, and part of their fear was tied up with what other people thought about them. Peter, particularly, in his reflections was clear that he still experienced fear in 'certain situations that I shouldn't'.[61] The morally judgemental tone of his comment implied that he perceived this as his own failing. Similarly, both Ken and Jeff described their experiences within a paradigm of individual failure to cope, rather than factoring in any wider organisational, economic or social contributory considerations. This is especially notable when all three effectively became stressed partly because of difficulties in dealing with and managing other people. For Ken and Peter, it was directly related to their supervisory role and for Jeff, it was not just about managerial responsibility for staff but also the problem-solving required in dealing with parents and pupils. Yet their descriptions of what happened and how they felt clearly related their stress to their own shortcomings, revealing continuity with earlier conceptions of nervous conditions. This is again suggestive of the slow transition from popular, public discourse to private understanding as most of the newspaper coverage of stress was beginning to challenge this, identifying external factors as contributory, if not causative, of people's stress.

Conclusion

Driven by competition from the new technology of television, the post-war period saw newspapers increasingly featuring more private subjects than previously as a way of maintaining their readership. This meant that health-related stories began to appear more frequently and, particularly from the 1960s onwards, the subject of everyday mental health and stress. Such reporting reflected a changing society, but also maintained continuity in terms of the initial approach to stress. Early stories about stress tended to focus on elite groups who were perceived to be more susceptible, such as university students and business leaders, situating stress very plainly within the class structure of Britain. Stress was also framed as resulting from modern conditions, effectively pathologising people's responses to change, something that was by no means new, as the authors of self-help books in the early century had also made this case.

The focus on elite groups changed, however, in the early 1970s when a more common element of stress reporting was the fact that anyone could suffer from stress, although status difference was still maintained to some extent through suggestions about the superior coping capabilities of business executives. Alongside the reporting of stress, another frequently raised concern was the huge growth in prescriptions for drugs such as tranquilisers, not least Valium. Personal testimony certainly acknowledged that this was a common practice, despite its effects not always being particularly positive. Such testimony also implied the gendering of stress, as the three men whose accounts are examined in this chapter were all experiencing stress within the context of a specific post-war understanding of masculinity that did not recognise mental distress and thus made it hard for men to acknowledge stress and the fear that came with it.

At the same time, there were other continuities with earlier periods in the way that domestic stress was discussed, women's stress being situated within the home, as in the case of the IoD wives and housewives in tower blocks. However, a time lag is evident between the newspaper language of stress and the vernacular terminology which tended to continue to be based around the concept of nerves. This is clearly seen in the personal accounts of three men who experienced stress in the 1960s and 1970s. Largely the language they used relates to nerves and nervous breakdowns and there is clear evidence of them knowingly relabelling those experiences with the term stress when they told their stories in the late 1990s. That is not to say, however, that the transmission of terminology was unidirectional. As Watkins has argued, the processes involved in the popularisation of medical and scientific ideas and the translation from expert to lay usage are complex.[62] However, my evidence suggests that while stress became the common term in media, medical and institutional discourse, people were slower to apply the term to themselves.

Despite the increased visibility of stress and discussion of its causes and sufferers in the media, personal experiences demonstrated that attitudes and understanding in everyday life were changing more slowly. The responses of colleagues to people's stress were at best sympathetic but lacking in understanding, and at worst dismissive and even suspicious. The privileging of physical models of health meant that the invisibility of a mental health problem rendered it non-existent to some who were wary of malingerers. Similarly, there was a pervasive assumption among sufferers as well as others that it was the individual's weakness that caused their stress, with little acknowledgement of external causation.

Overall, what the newspaper reporting and retrospective personal accounts of contemporary stress suggest is that the period from the late 1960s to the early 1980s was one of transition from a popular understanding that was based on a terminology of nerves and nervous breakdowns, to one that began to embrace stress as the more appropriate label for people's responses to a myriad of negative everyday experiences. It also transformed that understanding from privileging the susceptibility of specific elites to stress to viewing people of almost all ages, classes and occupations as potential 'victims of stress'.[63] As the next chapter will show, with this idea of victimhood came significant shifts in ideas about personal and organisational responsibility, stoicism and vulnerability.

Notes

1 Mills, Interview 1998.
2 David Kynaston, *Modernity Britain: Opening the Box, 1957–1959* (London; New York: Bloomsbury Publishing, 2013), p. 220.
3 Mills, Interview 1998.
4 'Keep Pools a Hobby – Not Worry Says Doctor', *Daily Mirror* (31 December 1953), p. 4.
5 '"Early Warning" Plan for Swots', *Daily Mirror* (16 July 1963), p. 10.
6 The *Daily Mirror* was Britain's largest circulation newspaper with sales of 4.5 million newspapers each day. Dilwyn Porter, '"City Slickers" in Perspective: The Daily Mirror, Its Readers and Their Money, 1960–2000',

Media History 9, 2 (1 August 2003): p. 141, https://doi.org/10.1080/13688800306758.

7 Bingham, *Family Newspapers?* pp. 2–3.

8 *Ibid.*, p. 20.

9 *Ibid.*, pp. 11–12.

10 Healy, *Prozac*, p. 6.

11 Watkins, 'American Vernacular', p. 52; Viner, 'Putting Stress in Life', pp. 399–400.

12 'The Boss and the Deadly 10lb', *Daily Mirror* (25 November 1960), p. 16.

13 Tredgold, *Human Relations* (1963), p. 127.

14 Watkins, 'American Vernacular', p. 57.

15 'Status Symbol of Stress and Strain', *Guardian* (16 March 1960), p. 7.

16 *Ibid.*

17 'A Boss's Burden Begins at Home', *Daily Mirror* (2 May 1968), p. 7.

18 *Ibid.*

19 'The Fright of Our Lives', *Daily Mirror* (10 October 1961), p. 11.

20 Joanna Bourke, *Fear: A Cultural History* (London: Virago, 2005), pp. 261–3.

21 'Advice on Problems of Middle-Age', *Daily Mirror* (14 June 1965), p. 5.

22 Ash, *Nerves in Order*, pp. 8–9.

23 Jackson, *Age of Stress*, pp. 192–3; Watkins, 'American Vernacular', pp. 61–2.

24 'The Seven Ages of Stress', *Daily Mirror* (20 October 1972), p. 25.

25 *Ibid.*; 'Status Symbol of Stress and Strain', p. 7.

26 Vernon Coleman, 'Stress: You Can't Escape It ... but Here's How You Can Enjoy It', *Daily Mirror* (12 December 1978), p. 9.

27 'Stress: The Big Danger to Your Health', *Daily Mirror* (9 July 1976), p. 21.

28 *Ibid.*

29 'Study Finds Stress Hits Workers Most', *Guardian* (29 February 1988), p. 3.

30 'Death on the Dole ... the New Threat', *Daily Mirror* (27 August 1980), p. 6.

31 *Ibid.*

32 MOA 'Work', H909.

33 'Replies to Spring Directive Social Well-Being' (1984), MOA, University of Sussex, H275.

34 Jackson, *Age of Stress*, p. 188.

35 Thomson, *Psychological Subjects*, p. 266.

36 'Fear!' *Daily Mirror* (18 September 1940), p. 4.

37 Jackson, *Age of Stress*, p. 145.
38 Claire Weekes, *Self-Help for Your Nerves* (Sydney; London: Angus & Robertson Ltd, 1963), p. 1.
39 For example: Claire Weekes, *Hope and Help for Your Nerves* (New York: Coward-McCann, 1963); Claire Weekes, *Peace from Nervous Suffering* (London: Angus and Robertson, 1972); Claire Weekes, *Self Help for Your Nerves* (London: Fontana, 1992).
40 Ronald Arthur Baxter Rorie, *Do Something about Those Nerves* (London; New York: Wingate Baker, 1969), p. 32.
41 *Ibid.*, p. 7.
42 'Drugs – Are They a Help or a Menace?' *Daily Mirror* (19 September 1955), pp. 6–7.
43 'Secrets of the Pill-Takers', *Daily Mirror* (20 September 1955), p. 9.
44 Callahan and Berrios, *Reinventing Depression*, p. 110.
45 P. A. Parish, 'The Prescribing of Psychotropic Drugs in General Practice', *Journal of the Royal College of General Practitioners* 92, supplement 4 (1971): p. 5.
46 *Ibid.*, pp. 7, 44.
47 Horwitz, *Anxiety*, pp. 120–2.
48 Edward Shorter, *Before Prozac: The Troubled History of Mood Disorders in Psychiatry* (Oxford; New York: Oxford University Press, 2009), p. 4.
49 Healy, *Prozac*, p. 226.
50 'Taking the Pain out of Strain', *The Times* (24 January 1985), p. 25.
51 Healy, *Prozac*, p. 6.
52 Haggett, *Male Psychological Disorders*, pp. 1–2.
53 Ken Duckworth, Mental Health Testimony Archive, 11 March 1999, C905/21/01, British Library Sound Archive.
54 *Ibid.*
55 M. G. Marmot et al., 'Health Inequalities among British Civil Servants: The Whitehall II Study', *The Lancet* 337, 8754 (1991): p. 1392, https://doi.org/10.1016/0140-6736(91)93068-K.
56 Peter Allen, Millennium Memory Bank Collection, 11 October 1998, C900/07016, British Library Sound Archive © BBC.
57 *Ibid.*
58 Mills, Interview 1998.
59 *Ibid.*
60 Michael Roper, *Masculinity and the British Organisation Man since 1945* (Oxford: Oxford University Press, 1994), p. 40.
61 Allen, Interview 1998.
62 Watkins, 'American Vernacular', p. 49.
63 'When the Floundering Has to Stop', *Guardian* (10 October 1984), p. 14.

6

The 'ruthless years': burn-out and the paradigm of stress

'Mental stress seems to be worse these days and no-one is interested. Talking to people similar to myself I realise that at the present time there is more stress than I can ever remember.'[1] These words of a middle-aged woman working part-time as an egg-grader on a farm in 1984 reflected the increasing awareness of stress as a popular concept by the 1980s. For many people, stress seemed a logical response to the often-repeated idea that modern life was somehow more challenging than in earlier periods. Although this idea and its associated notion of rapid change has been raised in earlier chapters, and undoubtedly could be tracked back to the nineteenth century and perhaps earlier, she made her remark in a Britain that *was* undergoing significant political, economic, social and technological transformations, affecting the everyday lives of ordinary people.[2]

Her comment reflected a significant public discourse of work and stress, seen in newspapers, television and, increasingly during the late 1980s and 1990s, in the burgeoning stress management industry. This was a discourse in which increasing numbers of employees were at risk from 'burn-out' brought about by working under constant high levels of stress. She followed up her initial observation by adding, 'Our health may not be worse, we just feel worse.'[3] Her perceptive statement captured one of the significant changes in the way people understood stress, and health in general, at the end of the twentieth century: what mattered was how it made you feel. As her comment suggested, people's health might not be worse (indeed by most medical criteria the health of the public in Britain had improved exponentially across the century), but how people *felt* about their health had altered considerably and much greater weight was being given to emotional responses and psychological well-being. A culture of 'emotional determinism' was developing that focused on the response of the individual to the pressures of everyday life, pathologising previously routine experiences, and leading to widespread acceptance of a sense of victimhood.[4] While this placed much greater weight on the role of external factors in causing stress, it also effectively undermined the agency of the sufferer and rendered them powerless in the face of their stressful circumstances. It also had repercussions for employers who might now find themselves held accountable for the stress that had previously been seen as the employee's responsibility.

This chapter explores how organisations were slow to formally recognise employee stress and reluctant to acknowledge its relationship to work and working conditions, despite the public discourse of stress in the 1980s and the growth of a stress management industry, largely focusing on stress in the workplace. By examining evidence from Lloyds Bank's internal and employee communications about stress, I illustrate the significant change in organisational stance from a 1980s managerial scepticism about employee stress to the development of a comprehensive package of stress management measures and messages by the late 1990s. While evidently not representative of all British organisations, this example from a large, national employer serves to illustrate the general trend during the period where other large organisations such as the Civil Service were also beginning to take heed of stress, with the Civil Service College introducing its first one-day senior management training course on managing stress in 1984.[5] Individual contemporary testimonies from MOP illustrate the frustrations of employees who sought help or support from their employers and colleagues during this period and highlight not only the extent of self-diagnosis of stress, but also the developing narrative of victimhood that by the late 1990s would overturn the previously received wisdom that stress was a problem of the individual and would instead lay the problem much more squarely at the feet of employers, with significant financial consequences.

These accounts show how the concept of stress was increasingly adopted and applied to personal circumstances as a way of explaining individual responses to the changing social and economic environment of late twentieth-century Britain. The parallel development of the so-called 'stress industry' contributed to a shift which initially saw stress management as the prerogative of high-status employees but swiftly evolved to incorporate a wider range of workers, although most were still white-collar employees, which was consistent with earlier constructions linking nerves with social status.[6] However, by the end of the twentieth century, stress was ubiquitous: it was part of the everyday discourse of working life; it was the reason for considerable absenteeism; it was the response to the challenge of change and continuity in gender roles. Everyone knew what stress was and most people believed that they experienced it at least some of the time.

Stress and work

In 1984 the recently re-established MOP asked its panel of respondents about their social well-being. This included a scaled response questionnaire and some open questions about health. Although not asked directly about stress, several wrote about recent experiences of it. A comprehensive school teacher explained, 'In the last month I have been prescribed mild tranquiliser [sic] as the doctor says I am suffering from "stress". I do not normally feel ill and do not normally feel particularly stressed.'[7] Another teacher explained his response to having pains in his chest: 'I went to the Doctor – he advised that I spent less energy on my teaching work. As a result I resigned from a number of committees I was on, reorganised my time so that I did my marking and preparation over a longer period. Overall I do now feel less tense and "strung up" about my work.'[8] Meanwhile, a local newspaper editor reported, 'I think my health is declining slowly – very slowly but perceptibly. Don't know if this is just advancing age or as a result of stress from my job. It seemed to start when I was promoted.'[9] These accounts are illustrative of the ways in which stress was being adopted by individuals to explain their own experiences, albeit with some hesitancy about new terminology indicated by their use of speech marks around the word stress. Such marks might also indicate some residual reluctance to acknowledge a mental health problem as the first writer was keen to point out that 'normally' she was not stressed. Similarly, the use of 'strung up' in inverted commas in the second account indicates recognition of employing a vernacular euphemism for stress, perhaps in preference to more medical language.

It is pertinent that although the questionnaire did not ask about stress, instead mentioning 'nervousness and tenseness' and asking whether respondents felt 'under strain', those answering the question-naire chose to use the term themselves. Although only answered by a few hundred people, the responses they gave in highlighting stress as the result of negative experiences suggest that people were responding differently to such events than they had done in the past. Indeed, what might previously have been ignored, endured or disguised by a physical proxy, was now labelled 'stress'. It was now becoming acceptable to recognise one's stress and seek advice and treatment from a doctor and to be relatively open about it. Asking for help rather than coping stoically alone was becoming the norm. In the third account, it is also pertinent that what might once have been seen as part of the inevitability of ageing was now attributed to stress, and specifically to the stress of increased work responsibilities. These examples of people talking about their stress demonstrate the ways in which people were taking up the terminology of stress to explain a range of work-related ills. Their highlighting of the term implies recognition of its newness and a certain tentativeness in applying it to themselves but also indicates the pathologising of experiences previously considered simply as elements of everyday life.

Popular discourse

The adoption of stress terminology occurred against a backdrop of news reporting that increasingly associated stress with particular professions. A *Sunday Times* article in 1987 stated that according to a conference organised by the Association of Assistant Masters and Mistresses, stress was forcing teachers into early retirement. The conference was told that at a school in Liverpool where seventy-three teachers were supposed to take part in a health day, twenty of them had such high blood pressure and stress-related problems that they were advised not to participate in the fitness exercises. A contributing problem was the attitude of head teachers who, the paper reported, were 'unsympathetic to stress among their staff, seeing it as a sign of weakness'.[10] Such an approach was certainly consistent with organi-sational policies across the century. However, less than a year later the newspaper's daily edition was reporting that 'thousands of head teachers are still queueing up for early retirement, with the occupation accepted as a "burn-out" profession', such evidence suggesting that many head teachers were perhaps simply too stressed themselves to understand and deal with their struggling subordinates.[11]

The term 'burn-out' was originally a colloquial description of the effects of chronic drug abuse but was adopted in the 1970s by Herbert Freudenberger, a US psychiatrist working in free clinics.[12] He used it to describe how working in care-giving and service occupations where the work was characterised by 'emotional and interpersonal stressors', could lead to 'overwhelming exhaustion, feelings of cynicism and detachment from the job, and a sense of ineffectiveness and lack of accomplishment'. Burn-out was a 'psychological syndrome in response to chronic interpersonal stressors on the job'.[13] Such human services organisations originated in the counter-culture of the 1960s and were intended to bring about social change through caring for the often-marginalised elements of society. What Freudenberger and others, such as social psychologist Christine Maslach, proposed as a solution to burn-out was a reversal of focus. Rather than concentrate on the needs of clients, as was the underlying ethos of human services, workers should instead focus on their own individual needs. Thus, the drive for social change became subordinated to the need for self-help, self-care and self-protection.[14]

By the 1980s in Britain the 'caring' professions, including teaching, were often constituted in the same way as Freudenberger's human services organisations. While such professions by no means constituted the elite understood previously to be the main sufferers of stress, nevertheless people in these professional roles were now perceived as more at risk. Newspaper reports frequently employed the idea of 'burn-out' as a way of emphasising the stressful nature and ultimately damaging effects of these jobs. For example, *The Times* quoted a study of five hundred senior nurses that found 85 per cent 'felt that they were overloaded at work' and concluded that nursing had 'high rates of sickness absence with high staff turnover compared with that for teachers and social workers', with the result that nursing careers were ending in 'disillusionment and burn-out'.[15] An earlier survey of hospital and family doctors in the same newspaper had quoted 83 per cent claiming they 'suffered periods of physical emotional or intellectual exhaustion'.[16]

Arguably, such reporting about stressed public sector workers was being used to highlight the changes to public services being made by a Conservative government intent on the free market and a smaller state. This focus on increasing stress in the public sector was occurring at a time of considerable transformation in relations between workers, employers and governments, where the broad post-war consensus about job security was giving way to unemployment, huge technological change and the casualisation of the workplace. The reduction in the power of the trade unions brought about through incremental legislation under Thatcher's government in the 1980s, and reinforced through the decline in manufacturing and consequent reduction in trade union membership, made the workplace an increasingly individualised space.[17] The emphasis was shifting from collective action to individual responsibility, and arguably this not only gave stress currency as a means of expressing dissatisfactions and fears about the changing workplace, but also provided an explanation for the experience of diminished collective support and collegiality that many workers were encountering.[18]

Many newspaper articles drew on the rapidly expanding field of academic research into work and stress, particularly that of Dr Cary Cooper, Head of the Business School at UMIST and 'one of the most vociferous and prolific stress researchers' of the time.[19] Cooper's work was quoted in numerous newspaper articles during the 1980s and 1990s and he appeared as a presenter and guest in various television programmes related to stress, one of the earliest a five-part series on Channel Four entitled 'How to survive the 9 to 5', broadcast in 1986. His stress league table of occupations published in the *Sunday Times* in 1985 listed sixty occupations from the most to least stressed, naming miners, police and construction workers at the head and museum workers and librarians at the bottom of the list, much to the consternation of some librarians. To be stressed was seen by some as validation of their hard work and the suggestion that a role was not stressful somehow undermined its status.[20] Key to Cooper's message was the fact that British organisations were losing money through their failure to address employee stress because of its impact on productivity and absenteeism. However, it was a message that British industry appeared reluctant to accept.

Organisational perspective

In 1983 T. F. H. Cullum, the General Manager of the Personnel Division of Lloyds Bank, wrote a memo to the Deputy Chief General Manager,

R. R. Amos, alerting him to an emergent issue raised by the Managers' Committee of the Lloyds Bank Group Staff Union (LBGSU): 'You will be aware of the growing concern by the public in recent years about the so-called increased stress which is apparently afflicting people in all walks of life.' His choice of words carefully indicated his own scepticism about the topic. Despite his apparent reservations, he went on to acknowledge that 'some of our 3,000 managers do suffer from stress, as evidenced by their medical symptoms', but also stated that 'the work situation is often only one element and that in many instances none of us knows anything about the personal home circumstances, or indeed over-indulgence in alcohol, etc., of those who claim to be over-stressed'. Notably, Amos underlined this latter sentence once, and the word 'claim' three times.[21] Notwithstanding the acknowledgement that stress *was* an issue for the organisation, there was evidently still a strong degree of resistance to the idea that it was work which created stress, and a decided inclination to ascribe causation to the individual and domestic factors rather than to employment.

The memo went on to suggest that there was a cohort of managers at a particular grade, aged 'at least 50', who were 'finding themselves possibly inadequate' and Cullum reported that in conversations with Partridge, the General Secretary of the LBGSU, it had transpired that this cohort were most often in contact with the union. Cullum concluded that those who had achieved higher levels of appointment than this group had done so because of their ability to 'control those elements which others, less capable, find stressful'. Thus, having explained to his own satisfaction that it was the flawed capabilities of certain unfortunate managers that were at the heart of the problem, he went on to propose a limited course of action.

Dealing with stressed managers was apparently the responsibility of the Regional General Managers (RGMs) to whom they reported, and problems 'could be headed off at an early stage if Managers felt able to talk openly to their Regional General Managers'. Unfortunately, as the memo then acknowledged, this did not often happen due to the fear among managers that such a discussion would leave them labelled inadequate or expose them to disciplinary action. Equally unhelpful was the fact that some of the RGMs were seen to be 'particularly unapproachable and unsympathetic to personal problems'. Concluding his memo, he noted that, unfortunately, he would be away on holiday when the next meeting with RGMs was due, so proposed writing to counsel them about how they and their teams should behave in relation to stress. Amos agreed this, although his handwritten reply on the memo also concurred with the assessment of RGMs and indicated some doubt as to the efficacy of a letter. He noted that personal qualities of sympathy and understanding were important, but that these either came 'naturally or not at all', concluding that 'in some cases no amount of tuition will help'.

Lloyds was one of the 'big four' high street banks of the 1980s and representative of large white-collar employer organisations undergoing considerable technological change. It also exemplified the changing corporate landscape of the 1980s and 1990s, including a series of public flotations in the financial services sector that drove a focus on share-holder value resulting in a series of mergers and acquisitions, which in turn required a succession of upheavals and reorganisations for employees.[22] The memo highlights the contradictory forces that were at work within Lloyds at the time, and was representative of many other similar contemporary organisations. On the one hand, there was understanding among both senior management and union repre-sentatives that growing awareness of stress both inside and outside the organisation was beginning to have an impact, but on the other, there was also significant organisational scepticism about stress itself and particularly its causation, and an apparent unwillingness, therefore, to take tangible action. Indeed, the attitudes revealed in the memo suggest considerable continuity with earlier conceptions of stressed or nervous workers whose suffering was attributed to inherent weakness rather than the nature of their work, working environment or organi-sational policies and practices. In the case of Lloyds Bank, experiences of stress were explained as resulting from the inability of certain managers to deal with stressful situations or the inadequate supervision or counsel of RGMs with poor interpersonal skills. It was the inadequa-cies of certain people rather than their work itself which was causing them to struggle.

The senior management of Lloyds Bank was by no means alone in its cautious and reluctant approach to acknowledging employee stress. Respondents to several MO directives in the 1980s and 1990s reported their own experiences of stress and the support or lack thereof from employers and colleagues. A thirty-four-year-old computer programmer suffering from stress due to overcrowded working conditions, a micro-managing supervisor, a terminally ill parent and pregnant wife reported experiencing significant physical symptoms such as 'waking up every morning knotted into a foetal position' and suffering from muscle pains and numb fingers. However, when he approached his personnel department, apart from listening sympathetically, they could not offer 'any advice other than to apply for another job elsewhere in the office'. He did this but found that having to start a new job simply compounded his stress.[23] Similarly, a Huddersfield teacher explained that 'The "Personnel" department may as well not exist in terms of stress counselling, career counselling or support of any description for a member of its workforce who is patently very ill and unable to function.'[24] Certainly, some employees felt that their stress had not only been caused by their work, but also that their suffering was either ignored or dismissed by employers.

In 1994 the *Guardian* reported that John Walker, an ex-social worker, had made legal history when a High Court judge ruled that his employers, Northumberland County Council, were liable for damages because their failure to provide a safe working environment had led to the nervous breakdown that ended his career. This was not the first time that stress had featured in a court case: a *Guardian* headline in 1974 reported the claim that a man was 'broken by stress' and that this led him to shoot four people.[25] However, the 1994 case placed stress firmly within the context of the workplace, and the ruling held that the Council had been 'in breach of its duty of care', which the newspaper explained put stress 'on the same footing as work accidents or industrial diseases'.[26] To some extent such a ruling was a logical outcome of the introduction of the Health and Safety at Work Act in 1974 and creation of the Health and Safety Executive to enforce its provisions, as these had placed a greater focus on the work environment and introduced greater organisational responsibility for employee well-being, mental as well as physical. Unsurprisingly, in the face of such a ruling, from the mid-1990s onwards many organisations began to put in place stress management and prevention measures. It was one thing to be told that stress affected productivity and thus the bottom line, but quite another to contemplate the levels of compensation paid out to workers like John Walker, who ultimately settled out of court for £175,000.[27]

Certainly by 1998 such moves were underway at Lloyds (by then Lloyds TSB). Its staff magazine *Frontrunner* announced in March that staff were to be surveyed about stress to aid in planning the organisation's Employee Support Strategy. The resulting letters about experiences of stress ran in the monthly publication for the next three issues, one anonymous employee writing, 'The sheer pace of change in TSB Business Banking over the last 12 months is much more than I have ever before experienced. I know that I don't speak just for myself when I say that the resulting levels of pressure and stress are excessive.' He or she went on to suggest that the organisation did not need to carry out a survey to find out what put people under pressure, and listed lack of human resources, experience and training, ever-increasing targets with fewer resources, competition among senior management, pace of change, overload of information and poor communication, as causes. It is pertinent that the writer explained, 'Personally, I would be too proud to seek counselling, preferring to face up to the situation in consultation with my line manager', although admitting that the 'local response may not be the best'.[28] Seemingly little had changed among the ranks of managers since the memo discussions about RGMs a decade earlier. This letter was followed up in following months by two further anonymous letters, praising the first writer for courage in voicing the view of many and offering further specific examples of causes of employee stress. These again included competition among senior managers to have the best results, with concomitant pressure passed down in increased workload to more junior staff.[29]

The fact that speaking out about stress was perceived as courageous by employees would appear to indicate that the concerns voiced in 1983 about managers' fears of being labelled inadequate or disciplined for poor performance were still a significant employee concern. The final part of this extended discussion in the Letters page of the magazine came in a response from the departing Managing Director of Business Banking, John Spence, who acknowledged the pace and quantity of change occurring while pointing out that 'there is no evidence of widespread stress-related absenteeism'.[30] This was a somewhat disingenuous response, for such evidence certainly might be hard to find if employees were nervous of admitting their stress. It was not uncommon, particularly among men, for experiences of psychological distress to be hidden behind physical symptoms.[31] Thus employees were much more likely to attribute absence to some physical proxy for stress, such as colds or digestive problems, as discussed in earlier chapters.[32] Potentially what this meant was that many employees were continuing to work despite their stress with the risk of storing up a latent body of medical problems which *would* eventually have a noticeable impact on absence statistics. Indeed, the fact that a year later the magazine featured an article about the launch of the organisation's guide to employee well-being benefits and support services, which included a confidential telephone counselling service and promised further communications about the development of support for stressed staff including the introduction of new stress awareness training, suggests that, statistics notwithstanding, there was now an organisational perception that the issue of stress needed to be addressed.[33] Arguably, the managerial ambivalence of the 1980s with its concern that employee stress might be an individual issue related to non-work factors or due to individual weakness was still present. However, by the late 1990s it was subordinate to concerns about compensation cases and the testimony of staff undergoing seemingly continuous change programmes resulting from mergers and acquisitions, technological change and the pressure to create shareholder value. While not all organisations in Britain were undergoing quite as much change as Lloyds TSB, nevertheless the issue of employee stress could no longer be ignored.

Managing stress

Although previous chapters have shown that there had been earlier research into and attempts to deal with and manage the symptoms of 'nervous workers' or sufferers of 'industrial neurosis', it was not until the 1980s and 1990s that a significant body of stress experts and stress management organisations began to appear in Britain, as what Patmore has labelled the 'stress industry' rapidly expanded.[34] The whole notion of 'managing' stress reflected the pathologisation of everyday experiences as something that needed to be avoided, prevented or treated. While a body of experts available to provide advice and guidance was indicative of the increase in service industries in Britain's changing economy. Initially, the stress industry targeted the high-status workers of the City, *The Times* reporting in 1987 on an apparently pioneering organisation which while offering health screenings was also 'teaching executives techniques on how to forestall post "Big Bang" stress' resulting from the deregulation of the City the previous year.[35] It also featured the work of Dr David Lewis, the founder of the 'Stress Watch' charity and provider of £2,000-a-day seminars for banks and other large companies, aimed at helping employees learn how to 'maximise their creative stress potential'. Dr Lewis's focus was not on stress avoidance, but on stress control through relaxation techniques and the keeping of a 'stress diary'. This would help employees to identify and learn from their peak performance days, which according to him, occurred when the stress balance was just right.[36] Such an approach was based on an understanding that some stress was necessary and indeed could have a positive effect on human functioning. Existing providers of business education and training with close ties to large organisations also entered into stress management, such as Ashridge Management College, which was reported to be offering a new 'Lifestyle planning for performance' programme in 1996. Its creator John Neal, fitness coach to the Middlesex Cricket Club and a consultant to several businesses, explained that lifestyle planning was 'for people who want to live beyond 60' and to avoid burn-out. For £600 participants received a day-and-a-half programme including discussions, modules on diet and exercise, stress management, time management, assertion and aggression training and prioritisation, as well as a physical fitness screening. Borrowing from US statistics, Neal claimed that British organisations were ignoring potential improvements in turnover, absenteeism and performance by failing to address lifestyle planning.[37] It is significant that despite a popular discourse which recognised that stress was something which anyone could suffer from, the organisations and programmes being reported in *The Times* (and other newspapers) as offering help were largely addressing the problem as an issue of the elite of senior managers and City workers. Undoubtedly, this was because the organisations which were offering these services were more likely to achieve their not inconsiderable fees by targeting the kinds of companies which could afford them. Inevitably, these were large corporates which employed high-flying executives who were both expensive to replace, therefore worth keeping healthy, and who might expect targeted stress management seminars as part of the package of benefits concomitant with their perceived work status. However, such employees were a tiny minority of the overall British workforce and therefore, among the wider ranks of the stressed, most people had to rely on their own efforts to deal with their work-related stress.

The computer programmer encountered earlier struggling with an overcrowded office, micro-managing supervisor and unhelpful personnel department, reported that although during that period of excessive stress he did not take time off work or visit his GP, if he were to experience such stress again he would go 'straight to the doctor'.[38] His response suggests a realisation that however much he might wish to be self-sufficient and stoic, he now appreciated that he could not cope alone, and did not need to. Such an admission is revealing of attitudes that were gradually reframing stress sufferers as victims of their environment and circumstances, rather than inherently weak individuals, and this reframing made help-seeking behaviour both acceptable and expected. Increasingly a visit to their GP was how people responded to stress, and several respondents told MO in 1984 that such visits had resulted in prescriptions for tranquillisers, with one man complaining bitterly about his subsequent addiction to Valium.[39] However, others found their GPs less than compliant in doling out prescription drugs. A twenty-nine-year-old woman explained that she had asked for tranquillisers during a 'particularly trying time' but 'was made to feel mine was a very frivolous request. I often wonder who the thousands of women are who are given tranquillizers and sleeping pills we all read about. Certainly no-one in my acquaintance, more's the pity.'[40]

In the absence of drugs, people turned to remedies that would have been instantly recognisable to the self-help authors of Chapter 1. There was no question of trying to carry on without some form of response, however simple. A retired machine tool operator explained that walking in the countryside and breathing fresh air without the feeling that someone was '"on my back" asking for more production' had a beneficial effect on his stress.[41] Others were still adhering to the benefits of tobacco advocated by Loosmore in 1920, despite awareness of its health dangers, for, according to one man, pipe smoking was 'good for the nervous system: it is impossible to be neurotic and smoke a pipe satisfactorily'.[42] A woman in her sixties reported turning to cigarettes when she was stressed, although she admitted that 'no doubt it is all in the mind about them soothing the nerves' and reflected that what was helpful was the distraction smoking offered from the 'frenzy that was building up'.[43] Other less malign remedies from earlier self-help sources were also still actively being used by sufferers from stress; for example, a seventy-two-year-old ex-secretary reported herself very satisfied with a self-help book titled *Relax and Live* which she had found in a second-hand bookshop. This included exercises she carried out to counter her tension and had proved so successful that she had been able to wean herself off a twelve-year Valium addiction.[44] A part-time auxiliary teacher who struggled for two years to get a clear diagnosis for her tension and depression, succumbing ultimately to tranquillisers and complete rest, reported finding a recording by Dr Claire Weekes which 'described my symptoms on a tape called nervous exhaustion'. With the aid of the recording, she was able to slowly recover her health, and avoid the overwork and worry which had triggered her original illness.[45]

Other sufferers claimed to keep their stress at a low level through diet, a retired author explaining, 'eat sensibly i.e. never over-eat, plenty of undercooked veg; little meat; vitamin tablet, often with iron, each day, skimmed milk, decaffeinated coffee, low fat, white bread – occasional chocolate and cream, few biscuits, tinned fruit, wine'.[46] Apart from the vitamins and decaffeinated coffee, her diet might have fitted well with those recommended in the self-help books of the interwar period. Such self-management also reflected contemporary dietary fads and reinforced a sense of agency against a condition that had no evident and simple cure. A middle-aged housewife felt she was better able to cope with her stress because of group therapy in the 1970s, although such mention of therapy was rare among MOP's respondents.[47] Another housewife told of the stress caused when her son's ship was sunk during the Falklands War of 1982 but explained that on discovering he had survived she made a conscious decision to change her life, enrolling in evening classes and volunteering in a charity shop. The result of these purposeful activities was that she felt 'fulfilled and much better in general health. Much less twitchy and depressed.'[48] Again, her choice to engage in occupations which interested her and distracted her attention was consistent with much of the early self-help advice discussed in previous chapters. Arguably, those suffering from stress relied on self-treatments which had changed little over the course of the century, unless their GP was willing to prescribe tranquillisers such as Valium. People might be much more aware and able to label their experiences as stress, but there were seemingly few new means of treating them.

However, not everyone perceived stress or the pressure and tension associated with it as negative. Cultural trends in the 1980s and 1990s could also be seen to lionise the thrusting go-getters of the new economy, symbolised by the power suit and mobile telephone, working long hours in high-powered roles and visible in popular Hollywood films such as *Wall Street* and *Working Girl*.[49] The characters in such entertainments were portrayed as apparently thriving in their high-pressure, stressful worlds of work. Similarly, the director of a large financial organisation told MOP in 1998, 'I thrive on stress – it is the most vivid colour in my life and I court it.' He believed that 'my old friend tension will keep me going many years, with luck' and suggested that if stress were absent from his life then 'senility will be just around the corner'.[50] He deliberately sought out stress, pursuing high-adrenaline hobbies such as riding a 'spirited horse, my high-powered bike' and public speaking and performing on stage. It was not only senior managers who acknowledged that some stress could be advantageous, as a cleaner and barmaid commented, 'I've always found that I work better under pressure even at work the busier we are the better I like it.'[51] However, their views were exceptions rather than the norm, and what was critical in these cases was both their awareness of their stress and, particularly in the case of the director, his deliberate approach to managing it. He explained, 'I drink alcohol. At times I have considered giving this up, but I am convinced that it benefits me by relieving tension.' He also admitted that his wife's view was that he was hooked on adrenaline and therefore he needed alcohol to counter the rush he got from engaging in challenging work and risky and adventurous leisure pursuits. He admitted that without alcohol he would be 'ill from tension and stress'. Although his doctor may have wished him to find an alternative approach, he had found a way of both benefiting from the effects of stress and balancing them by relaxing through drinking alcohol.[52]

While his enjoyment of his stress was perhaps a little unusual, as Haggett has shown his use or overuse of alcohol as a coping mechanism was a common practice, particularly for men.[53] His experience reflects what seemed to be the paradox of stress: events and experiences that caused considerable stress for some people were taken in their stride, and even thrived on, by others. This was the point that caused scepticism at Lloyds Bank in the 1980s – how did some managers cope with the targets and competition which apparently so stressed a cohort of their colleagues? Why did some people feel stressed by experiences that others found merely challenging? The *Sunday Times* article mentioned previously reported three factors which his research maintained were critical to whether someone experienced work stress: lack of autonomy, a poor relationship with superiors and the dual-career family. Certainly at least one of these factors was consistent with the debate at Lloyds Bank in the early 1980s. The dual-career families factor was certainly on the rise during the period, the *Sunday Times* reporting that changes in the workforce now meant that two-thirds of women were in work.[54] Nevertheless, there were continuities as well as changes in the interactions between domestic and workplace stress.

Domestic stress

Earlier chapters have highlighted women's experiences of tension and stress related to working in the home, interpersonal relationships, issues of control of time and domestic resources. To a large extent, these continued to be common in the 1980s and 1990s. Echoing the suburban neurosis of the 1930s and the isolation of post-war council estates, a thirty-eight-year-old housewife explained to MO in 1984 that she had 'devoted my life to my children and home' and was wondering what was next for her. 'I am not a career-minded person and do not want to go back to office work were it available. Life has changed due to lack of transport from village to town and isolation creeps in and neuroses along with it.'[55] Similarly, a Kent housewife complained in terms which Flora Klickmann in the 1920s or Hannah Gavron in the 1950s would have recognised: 'I am a housewife with one son at school and I don't meet enough people. I suffer from stress which I think is due to not being "out in the world" enough. Housework is boring and repetitive but I would not want to go out to work while my son is small.'[56] The challenge of the housewife role and caring responsibilities was a perennial one, but it was increasingly complicated for many women by the newer demands of their own careers, the age-old difficulties of tricky family relationships and an ageing population of parents.

The results of such a balancing act could indeed be problematic. As an ex-nurse explained, 'I started with nervous trouble fifteen years ago and was in hospital for six weeks. This was caused by over anxiety about my husband's health, also pressure of work.'[57] A retired teacher explained that she too worried about her husband's health 'as he has to work very hard (one day off a fortnight and very long hours of shift work!)'. This put them both 'under a great deal of stress', which tended to make her health worse as she could 'see that he is often very tense and I worry in case he has a coronary'.[58] A middle-aged woman living in the West Midlands reported, 'Most people I know in full time employment, especially my husband, have to work far too hard and with enormous stress. He feels he has no time to rest, so a lot of my "spare" time is spent in trying to relieve this stress, going for walks etc.' She had already given up some of her own work as an adult education teacher due to 'a very stressful period', but now managing her husband's stress was impinging on the 'spare' time she had claimed back, and had become part of her domestic workload and a potential contributor to her own stress.[59] These three cases demonstrate the pervasive nature of work-related stress, brought into the home through the husband's experience, but creating similar suffering in wives as they worried about or tried to counter the effects of stress on their husbands. They were not alone in such concerns, as *The Times* reported in 1991, quoting a survey of chief executives and their spouses. It found that 62 per cent of the latter believed work overload was a source of strain on their husbands and almost half believed 'job burn-out' was a real risk.[60]

However, worrying about and caring for husbands were not the only factors contributing to female stress, as a part-time secretary illustrated. Describing a situation which was becoming increasingly common, she commented that 'My general health is very good – my one problem is tension. I look after my elderly frail mother (85) who, although not living with me, takes up a great deal of my time. I am virtually trying to run two homes.'[61] Her account highlights a form of work stress associated not with paid employment, but with the considerable range of unpaid work performed by women within the domestic environment. While this was certainly not a new phenomenon at the end of the twentieth century, for childcare remained an ongoing challenge for many families, elderly relatives *were* living longer, often alone and at some distance from adult children and often with more complex medical care requirements. At the same time that employment opportunities were increasing for women, their caring responsibilities were also demanding time and attention involving many in a tricky balancing act which brought with it tensions and pressures which very often resulted in stress.[62] As one woman guiltily admitted, 'Sadly my father has just been admitted to a Nursing Home, but suddenly I have had the tension and stress removed from my life and have this wonderful feeling of being permanently on holiday.'[63] In addition, for some there was a growing sense that juggling domestic responsibilities and full-time work was not simply an aspiration but an expectation, illustrated in newspaper coverage of so-called 'have it all' superwomen like Nicola Horlick, who combined a high-earning City role with raising six children.[64]

For others, it was wider family dynamics that caused stress. As a fifty-year-old receptionist explained, 'My relationship with parents-in-law was always a great source of stress. Nothing seemed to please my mother-in-law. For the first 17 years of our marriage we had to visit them on a Sunday every fortnight without fail and spend the day with them from 11.00am to 6.30pm.' She explained that her husband insisted on this despite its effect on her: 'When I went back to work on the Monday I used to feel drained and stressed out right away. What with that and the stress from customers where I worked I often got run-down.'[65] The difficulties of dealing with the tensions arising from family relationships reduced her capacity to deal with her work-related stress. A part-time teacher from Cheshire reported that much of her stress came from family relationships, in particular, 'the relation-ship between me and my son (19) and the triangular relationship between him, me and my husband, his stepfather'.[66] The increased complexities of family structures resulting from higher rates of divorce in late twentieth-century Britain often created additional strain for women in their role as family mediator.[67] She went on to admit that to a great extent it was her attempts to second-guess causes of conflict in order to defuse them that created her stress, remarking that 'Ours is a fairly happy home environment and much of the stress I suffer is of my own making. But when my son is unhappy about something, or if he does something that I assume my husband will be unhappy about then I worry like hell and usually end up making myself feel awful.' Contrary to the previous account, her solution was work: 'to escape the stress I manage to aggravate at home I go to work. I am not a workaholic, and I can't say I really love my job, but it takes my mind off any worries at home.'[68]

Such accounts ran counter to the usual narrative of the work environment as the main cause of stress but reflected research reported in *The Times* in 1994 that argued that women who went out to work suffered 'markedly less anxiety, depression and minor ailments' compared to stay-at-home housewives. While the research sample had consisted of middle-class housewives with school-age children and no financial imperative to work, it had concluded that what they missed was the sense of achievement and support offered by the work environment.[69] For women their experience of stress often resulted from a complex interplay of domestic and work-related tensions that drew on established gender roles often relating to caring responsibilities. However, for those women not in paid employment outside the home there were strong continuities with earlier periods in terms of the tensions and stress arising from the housewife role, as discussed in earlier chapters. It was rarer for men to recount domestic causes of stress, although the thirty-four-year-old computer programmer mentioned earlier in the chapter did include his mother's terminal illness among the factors that had driven him to seek help. While women often explained their stress as a result of both domestic responsibilities and workplace troubles, many of the people who contributed to MOP during the 1980s and 1990s were clear that there were wider societal reasons for the increase in stress.

Causes of stress

Writing in 1997, a male charity worker explained, 'There are precious few jobs for life now. With a constant labour surplus, jobs will remain less secure than they did 25 years ago when there was almost full employment. I think this puts huge stresses on a lot of people.'[70] The fear of unemployment and the experience of being unemployed, both of which became more widespread because of economic recessions in the 1980s and early 1990s, were recognised as stress-inducing. A twenty-three-year-old man reported having 'a great deal of stress from being unemployed', although he hoped this was only a transient state.[71]

Even for those in employment, it seemed that the relationship between employee and employer had changed. As a female carer from Aberystwyth summed up in 1997, 'Very many people are employed on short term contracts so job security has gone.'[72] A primary school teacher explained,

'As the years have gone by and the job has changed and become increasingly stressful, I saw myself and indeed, planned to take early retirement
at 50 years of age.' Unfortunately, this was no longer an option thanks
to public sector policy changes and for her and her colleagues the thought
of carrying on until they were sixty was 'unbearable' and morale had
taken a 'nose-dive'.[73] These accounts reflect perceived changes in working
conditions in many industries that in turn affected attitudes towards
work and its potential to cause psychological harm. A retired social
worker blamed long hours for the increase in stress: 'It seems that now,
those in jobs have to work even longer hours, under more stress, and
with less security than we did. They often have greater financial reward
but less time in which to enjoy it.'[74] Her view was not unreasonable.
For although the period up to the late 1970s had seen working-time
requirements gradually reduce, between 1981 and 1991 many people's
hours of work grew, with households of two working adults completing
an additional six hours of work per week often coupled with a palpable
increase in work intensity.[75] Britain in the last decades of the twentieth
century was shifting rapidly to a service economy and with this came
new jobs and ways of working which carried their own potential for
stress. Work practices such as Human Resource Management, while
emphasising concepts such as team working and empowerment, in
many ways increased managerial surveillance and focused on individual
rather than team responsibility.[76] Other new approaches to work such
as Just-in-time Production and Total Quality Management intensified
the nature of work, while new technology enabled a long-hours culture,
where the lines between working and non-working time were beginning
to blur.[77]

Those working in the new call centre industry found themselves in
large, depersonalised offices where not only were the words they could
speak scripted, but the basic biological functioning of their bodies had
to fit to a carefully calibrated and regimented system of lavatory and
lunch breaks, all under the relentless demands of the automated call
management system. Part of the strain of such work came from the
emotional labour of performing specific employer-prescribed emotions
intended to create a particular experience for the customer, while
repressing their own natural emotional responses.[78] As a receptionist
from Preston working in a similar service role explained, 'Some people
get very angry and abusive both to your face and on the phone. You

have to be "nice" to people all the time and never get angry yourself even when they shout and swear at you.'[79] The *Guardian* reported in January 1999 that European Commission research into call-centre workers, the majority of whom were women, advised that they suffered 'burn-out' within six months and most left their jobs within a year due to the strain.[80]

While the expansion of the service industry in Britain undoubtedly increased the propensity for people to work in such conditions, emotional labour was not of itself a new phenomenon. What was new, however, was the way that people responded to such experiences. Comments from a couple of MOP respondents are suggestive. A medical secretary argued that 'There seems to be one over-riding factor in modern life which I am sure makes for neurosis and ill-health. It is the fact that one is always encouraged to seek help, from the vicar, social services, the doctor and Aunt Minnie on the woman's page.'[81] What is critical to her comment is the acknowledgement that the norm in the face of negative experiences was no longer stoicism and coping. The popular discourse of stress (indeed of health in general) encouraged help-seeking from experts. The individual was no longer deemed capable of dealing with their own emotional responses to the pressures and tensions of home or work life, and this undermining of personal agency effectively encouraged the pathologising of day-to-day life. This in turn was supported by a regular media diet of health and medical stories, as a comment from a thirty-year-old teacher revealed when she opined, 'Undoubtedly the media makes us more aware of our health and that is certainly true of myself now, whereas 5 years ago I never gave it a thought.'[82] Health-scare stories were an increasing feature of the media and, as the comment implies, encouraged a level of introspection about well-being and illness that in turn fostered a sense that stress was the normal response to the troubles of day-to-day life.

Arguably, two things came together during the last decades of the twentieth century. First, there was considerable societal and economic change: more women in the workforce; periods of high unemployment; and changing employment patterns that reduced security and no longer promised a job for life. Second, a greater focus on how one felt brought to the fore a growing awareness of the stresses and strains of life which popular discourse encouraged people to see in medicalised terms. Was working life harder? Were people more stressed? Within the context of the period and according to people's accounts of their experiences the answer would appear to be positive, even though in many ways conditions of work, living standards and rates of morbidity were vastly improved compared to only decades before. A greater awareness of personal well-being (or lack of well-being) meant that by the end of the twentieth century it could seem that stress was everywhere.

Conclusion

During the 1980s and 1990s the public discourse of stress, especially in newspapers, increasingly focused on employees in specific professions as particularly susceptible to stress and at risk from conditions such as 'burn-out'. This was aided by the expansion of organisations and experts ready and willing to provide support in stress management to both organisations and individuals, at a cost. Initially the focus of high-status workers and the bigger corporations, the 'stress industry' expanded during the period to enable organisations such as Lloyds Bank to move from a position of scepticism about employee stress in the mid-1980s to spending large sums on employee well-being pro-grammes that included stress management and counselling by the late 1990s. This change of corporate focus was driven partly by the need to comply with the ways in which the law was interpreting employer responsibilities under the Health and Safety Act, but also by the increasing expectations of employees themselves driven by the very public discourse of stress.

However, many organisations were slow to recognise employee stress despite increasing research suggesting its economic impact. The testimony of MOP respondents illustrates the frustrations of many employees who, with a new public awareness of stress, self-diagnosed their suffering but found little support when they sought help in the workplace. This helped to reinforce a growing sense of victimhood in which the stress sufferer was no longer suffering because of their own inherent weakness, but because external, often work-related circumstances had driven him or her to become stressed or even 'burned-out'. There was a validation in being stressed.[83] Recognising one's own stress and seeking medical help from one's GP became increasingly the norm, although many people relied on treatments which were much the same as those recommended in self-help books much earlier in the century. People were no longer willing to struggle on stoically and there was less stigma in being open about seeking help. Work stress often impinged on domestic life, and for women, their dual role as employee and domestic care-giver could both compound, but also sometimes alleviate stress. Strong continuities with earlier periods existed in terms of the tensions arising from the housewife role and the way in which male work stress was brought into the home and contributed to female anxieties. People increasingly used the concept of stress to explain their own psychological and physical responses to personal circumstances affected by the changing social and economic environment of late twentieth-century Britain. The result was that by the end of the century it seemed that no aspect of everyday life in Britain was exempt from the risk of stress: stress was now ubiquitous.

Notes

1 MOA 'Social Well-Being', S496.
2 Stephen Brooke, 'Living in "New Times": Historicizing 1980s Britain', *History Compass* 12,1 (2014): 22–3, https://doi.org/10.1111/hic3.12126.
3 MOA 'Social Well-Being', S496.
4 Füredi, *Therapy Culture*, pp. 6, 25.
5 'Civil Service College Annual Report and Accounts' (Cabinet Office, April 1984), The National Archives, p. 25.
6 Patmore, *Truth*, p. 47. Patmore challenges the whole concept of stress and particularly charges those advocating stress management (the 'stress industry') with doing more harm than good.
7 MOA 'Social Well-Being', B1187.
8 *Ibid.*, F198.
9 *Ibid.*, H722.
10 'Sir Calls It a Day as Pressure Builds', *The Sunday Times* (25 October 1987).
11 'Concern at Teachers Quitting "burn-out" Careers', *The Times* (1 June 1988), p. 2.
12 I am using 'burn-out' rather than 'burnout' as this is the form most often used in popular media coverage of the period in Britain.
13 Christina Maslach, Wilmar B. Schaufeli and Michael P. Leiter, 'Job Burnout', *Annual Review of Psychology* 52, 1 (2001): p. 399, https://doi.org/10.1146/annurev.psych.52.1.397.
14 Matthew J. Hoffarth, 'The Making of Burnout: From Social Change to Self-Awareness in the Postwar United States, 1970–82', *History of the Human Sciences* (2017), p. 42, https://doi.org/10.1177/0952695117724929.

15 '"Conspiracy of Silence" Is Blamed for Cost of Stress among Nurses', *The Times* (2 May 1986), p. 3.

16 '"Burn-out" Diagnosis on Hard-Pressed Doctors in NHS', *The Times* (10 March 1984), p. 3.

17 Anthony Seldon and Daniel Collings, *Britain under Thatcher*, Seminar Studies in History (Harlow: Longman, 2000), p. 69.

18 Melling, 'Labouring Stress', pp. 163–4.

19 Fiona Jones, Jim Bright and Angela Clow, *Stress: Myth, Theory and Research* (Harlow; New York: Prentice Hall, 2001), p. 7.

20 'Working Can Be a Health Hazard', *The Sunday Times* (24 February 1985), p. 7.

21 T. F. H. Cullum, 'Note for Mr R. R. Amos, Deputy Chief General Manager' (28 July 1983), HO/GM/Off/213, Lloyds Banking Group Archive.

22 For example, in 1995 Lloyds Bank acquired Cheltenham & Gloucester and merged with Trustee Savings Bank. See 'Our Heritage: Timeline', Lloyds Banking Group, www.lloydsbankinggroup.com/our-group/our-heritage/timeline/. Accessed 15 August 2016.

23 'Replies to Autumn 1998 Directive Staying Well and Everyday Life' (1998), MOA, University of Sussex, C2722.

24 'Replies to Summer 1997 Directive Doing a Job' (1997), MOA, University of Sussex, N1552.

25 'Man "Broken by Stress"', *Guardian* (13 June 1974), p. 6.

26 'Damages for Overwork', *Guardian* (17 November 1994), p. 1.

27 'Social Worker Wins £175,000 for Breakdowns', *Independent* (27 April 1996), p. 1.

28 Anonymous employee, 'Stress – Support, Not Survey', *Frontrunner* (March 1998), Lloyds Banking Group Archive, p. 2.

29 Anonymous employee, 'Well Said, and Thank You from All of Us!' *Frontrunner* (May 1998), Lloyds Banking Group Archive, p. 2.

30 John Spence, 'Response to Last Month's Letter from a TSB Business Banking Manager Concerning Stress at Work', *Frontrunner* (June 1998), Lloyds Banking Group Archive.

31 Haggett, *Male Psychological Disorders*, p. 11.

32 See Chapters 3 and 5.

33 'Some Tender Loving Care for Staff', *Frontrunner* (December 1999), Lloyds Banking Group Archive, p. 4.

34 Patmore, *Truth*, p. 1.

35 'Stressing Pressures', *The Times* (12 August 1987), p. 15.

36 'When the Going Gets Tough', *The Times* (29 November 1990), p. 22.

37 'Take Stress out of Success', *The Times* (6 June 1996), p. 23.

38 MOA 'Staying Well and Everyday Life', C2722.

39 MOA 'Social Well-Being', A0121.
40 *Ibid.*, I720.
41 *Ibid.*, L689.
42 *Ibid.*, D951. Loosmore, *Nerves*, p. 84.
43 MOA 'Social Well-Being', B058.
44 John Kennedy, *Relax and Live* (London: Prentice Hall, 1953). 'Social Well-Being', D153.
45 MOA 'Social Well-Being', M1013.
46 *Ibid.*, W627.
47 *Ibid.*, T1186.
48 *Ibid.*, T1152.
49 Oliver Stone, *Wall Street* (Twentieth Century Fox, 1987); Mike Nichols, *Working Girl* (Twentieth Century Fox, 1988).
50 MOA 'Social Well-Being', C110.
51 *Ibid.*, J742.
52 *Ibid.*, C110.
53 Ali Haggett, 'Gender, Stress and Alcohol Abuse in Post-War Britain', in Jackson (ed.) *Stress in Post-War Britain*, p. 51.
54 'Working Can Be a Health Hazard', p. 7.
55 MOA 'Social Well-Being', G218.
56 *Ibid.*, D1226.
57 *Ibid.*, W569.
58 *Ibid.*, M387.
59 MOA 'Staying Well and Everyday Life', C2654.
60 'One in Four Captains of Industry Wants to Jump Ship', *The Times* (15 April 1991), p. 3.
61 MOA 'Social Well-Being', S1089.
62 Roberts, *Women and Families*, p. 19.
63 MOA 'Social Well-Being', B044.
64 'Horlick Proves You Can Have It All', *Guardian* (24 July 1999), p. 1.
65 MOA 'Staying Well and Everyday Life', C1713.
66 *Ibid.*, E743.
67 'Divorces in England and Wales 2010', Office for National Statistics, 8 December 2011, www.ons.gov.uk/peoplepopulationandcommunity/births deathsandmarriages/divorce/bulletins/divorcesinenglandandwales/2011-12-08. Accessed 19 April 2016. Whereas in 1970 just over a fifth of marriages had ended in divorce by the 15th wedding anniversary, this figure had risen to one-third by 1995.
68 MOA 'Staying Well and Everyday Life', E743.
69 'Unhappy High-Flyers and Housewives under Stress', *The Times* (30 November 1994), p. 34.

70 MOA 'Doing a Job', G2701.
71 MOA 'Social Well-Being', H1291.
72 MOA 'Doing a Job', P1009.
73 *Ibid.*, N1552.
74 *Ibid.*, P2546.
75 Francis Green and Keith Whitfield, 'Employees' Experience of Work',
    in William Arthur Brown, Alex Bryson and Keith Whitfield (eds) *The
    Evolution of the Modern Workplace* (Cambridge: Cambridge University
    Press, 2009), p. 206.
76 Arthur McIvor, *Working Lives: Work in Britain Since 1945* (Basingstoke:
    Palgrave Macmillan, 2013), 197. Wainwright and Calnan, *Work Stress*,
    p. 136.
77 P. E. Waterson et al., 'The Use and Effectiveness of Modern Manufacturing
    Practices: A Survey of UK Industry', *International Journal of Production
    Research* 37, 10 (1999): p. 2273, https://doi.org/10.1080/002075499190761.
    Just-in-time Production was about 'making products in direct response
    to internal or external customer demands (rather than building in advance
    to maintain stock levels)', and Total Quality Management involved 'seeking
    continuous change to improve quality and making all staff responsible
    for the quality of their work'. For a brief discussion of their impact on
    workers see McIvor, *Working Lives*, pp. 230–1.
78 Arlie Russell Hochschild, *The Managed Heart: Commercialization of
    Human Feeling* (London: University of California Press Ltd, 1983), p. 7.
79 MOA 'Staying Well and Everyday Life', C1713.
80 'Phone Workers' "Brain Strain"', *Guardian* (6 January 1999), p. 5.
81 MOA 'Social Well-Being', D781.
82 *Ibid.*, M1327.
83 Füredi, *Therapy Culture*, pp. 177–8.

Conclusion

Working in the oil industry in Scotland in the 1970s, James Lyon started to have strange physical symptoms: 'I was violently sick going home in the car, for no apparent reason ... and then on another occasion, the same sort of thing happened, just out of the blue for no reason at all.' Speaking in a life history interview in 2003, he explained that he was working very long hours, 'three, four nights a week, weekends ... I just couldn't keep up with it.' Eventually, he went for a check-up 'and they reckoned it was nerves or something was affecting my stomach. It was actually overwork and stress and stuff like that.'[1] James' explanation appeared as part of a broader narrative about why he set up his own business. This was due to his frustrations with organisational inefficiencies that led to consistent and repeated expectations that employees would work evenings and weekends. Despite descriptions of the long hours he was working, and of problems within the organisation at the time, he did not connect his sudden physical symptoms with the pressures of work. He could acknowledge these physical ailments but did not recognise them as resulting from stress, even when they appeared to have no other apparent cause.

I have argued in this book that throughout the twentieth century, people often privileged physical symptoms and explanations over the psychological, or what they believed to be a mental health problem. They used such physical ailments, which were often related to the digestive system, as proxies for their stress, sometimes knowingly, but often unconsciously. While physical symptoms were obviously real, and in James' case were indeed related to his stomach, the tendency for much of the century was to focus simply on the treatment of the physical without too much questioning of its causation. This avoided any recognition of the psychological and any hint of mental health problems and hence stigma which might threaten employment or sense of self.

This avoidance also underpinned a very common belief within much popular, institutional and organisational understanding of stress, that causation was strongly linked to the individual's inherent weakness or predisposition, rather than their circumstances, environment or the demands placed upon them. Thus, James' admission about his work that he 'just couldn't keep up with it' made his inability the main problem, rather than the amount of work that was demanded of him or the conditions in which those demands came about. Although he initially failed to see the connection, his account did also directly identify work as the cause of his stress, but it illustrates the fact that the symptoms of stress did not always appear in the location that caused them, and that stress might arise from a complex interplay of work, domestic and personal factors. This led to stress very often being not only unacknowledged but unacknowledgeable. James' apparent inability to connect his overwork and his symptoms reflects a norm of coping and stoicism that, in the earlier part of the century particularly, often resulted from economic necessity and a survivalist approach that ensured that any stressful experiences had to go unacknowledged. Stoicism privileged suffering in silence and privacy and was the norm in the face of distress for much of the century. It was closely related to concepts of the self, duty and respectability that favoured self-reliance and coping. Thus, anything that threatened work, such as stress, was problematic beyond the simple experience of suffering. Having a nervous condition threatened a sense of self that was predicated on stoic resilience and the status that came with economic security. This helps to explain why people were very often either dismissive of their suffering or deliberately imprecise about it. Non-medical terminology enabled explanations about nerves, and nervous suffering particularly, to cover a multitude of conditions and allowed the sufferer to be vague about the seriousness of their condition, that is if they admitted to it at all.

During the Second World War, such stoicism became an inherent part of the ideology of the Home Front and underpinned much state propaganda. The public health leaflet 'Just Nerves!' did acknowledge the stress that the population was under, not just from the fear of bombing, but from the problems and frustrations arising from the relentless compromises and challenges of wartime living. However, in practice it offered little more than a rallying call for people to cope, get on with their wartime responsibilities and refrain from seeing their own suffering as in any way unique. It was only in the post-Second World War period with the development of a more affluent and educated population, with greater opportunities and expectations of both work and domestic life, that stoicism ceased to be the appropriate response, and experiences which previously were ignored could become problematised, in a way that contributed to the growth of the concept of stress.

The way that James explained his experience also exemplifies my argument that the 1970s was a decade of transition between the lexicon of nerves and the terminology of stress. He told his story in 2003 but was describing a period in the early 1970s and quite naturally used the language of the time, describing being diagnosed with 'nerves or something'. However, he immediately reinterpreted this explanation to a more contemporaneous description as 'stress and stuff like that'. The linguistic shift is significant in illustrating this transitional period in the popular understanding of stress. During the 1970s the popular discourse of stress saw an expansion of the categories of people who might be at risk of stress. However, while this was becoming more and more prevalent within popular and public discourse, it took somewhat longer for people to apply such conceptualisations to themselves, which also contributed to James' failure to recognise his own stress initially. James' explanation for his symptoms also revealed a desire for ambiguity. He labelled his experience as nerves 'or something' and then rephrased this to the contemporary term, 'stress', adding 'and stuff like that'. This suggests his own desire to leave the explanation for his experience fluid, perhaps as a means of denial because he was uncomfortable with the idea of mental ill-health or because it did not sit well with his sense of self. Both nerves and stress were popularly conceived as flexible terms that enabled the sufferer to avoid the specificity associated with other psychological diagnoses. 'Stuff like that' allowed the sufferer to situate their experience on a continuum, deciding for themselves, in different contexts, the weight they wished to give to their experience. James Lyon's experience and his account of it demonstrate some of the main arguments presented in this book about how stress was understood and explained during the twentieth century in Britain. More significantly, it reaffirms the focus of the book on the everyday experience of ordinary people and the factors that informed how they understood, interpreted and acknowledged the popular and vernacular concepts of nerves and stress that existed during the century.

Overall in this book, I have sought to address the question of what people suffered from before stress was available as a diagnosis, and how it came to be ubiquitous within British society by the end of the century. People adopt the ideas and labels which are socially and culturally acceptable at the time, and this applies to health and ill-health too. Thus, for much of the twentieth century, people's explanations of their nervous conditions or stress often privileged physical explanations and symptoms as these were both more acceptable and more acknowledgeable than psychological or psychiatric explanations. This was evident during the Second World War. MO research on absenteeism among conscripted workers, instead of acknowledging the psychological impact of wartime conditions, listed a range of minor illnesses that stood as proxies for the stress that undoubtedly arose in such challenging conditions.[2] It was the problems and frustrations arising from the relentless compromise and challenges of wartime living that had an impact on people's psychological well-being, as much as the fear and anxiety of bombings. Like James Lyon's experience at the beginning of this chapter, the case studies of stress in the 1970s examined in Chapter 5 also revealed people focused on physical symptoms and highlighted the scepticism which was very often the response from others when stress sufferers had no visible physical injury. Arguably, the privileging of physical symptoms helped to both disguise stress but could also validate suffering by presenting it as a more tangible ailment.

Before stress became the popular label for experiences of dealing with the troubles of life, the language of nerves and a multiplicity of synonyms for nerves and nervousness were how people explained their experiences. From a popular perspective there is a continuum of such experiences which in the early twentieth century might sit within the umbrella of neurasthenia and nerves and, by the end, that of stress. Although Selye's formulation of the stress concept and its subsequent redefinitions within medicine and psychology were based around specific, diagnostic explanations, popular understanding is, by its nature, always more general, and I maintain that people did not make the distinctions which doctors or other professionals might. The language and descriptions of symptoms in the popular sources, such as self-help books, MO writings, oral histories and film and newspapers, offered up a variety of descriptions and explanations which to my reading are analogous with our contemporary stress paradigm. Certainly, other scholars of culture and medicine have come to similar conclusions, acknowledging the affinities between concepts such as nerves, stress, strain and pressure.[3] However, some of the symptoms that suggest themselves as forerunners for stress might equally be claimed by those who equate some of the language of nerves with depression – such is the mutability of this grey area of human experience.[4] Certainly, in response to the claim that cases of depression had hugely increased by the end of the twentieth century, Callahan and Berrios argued that numbers of sufferers had hardly changed since the 1950s, but that depression was previously hidden behind other labels, with both formal medical diagnostic categories and vernacular usage contributing to this concealment.[5]

Throughout the twentieth century, there was a belief that modern life itself was becoming increasingly challenging to the psyche. Every decade of the century provides examples of concerns that technological, economic and social changes were increasing the pressure on people's everyday lives. While in the first half of the century in Britain technological developments such as telephony, radio, motor vehicles and cinema were blamed, later concerns focused on consumer culture, the digital industrial revolution and the conversion to an economy based on service industries rather than manufacturing. Broadly speaking, nerves and then stress were framed as an appropriate response to the difficulties and challenges that change brought across the century, within a society that increasingly privileged medical and psychological explanations. However, whether work-related or domestic and due to increased challenges of life or not, it was also largely understood, both popularly and institutionally, that nerves or stress resulted from an inherent weakness of the individual. It was their susceptibility or failure to cope with their life experiences, rather than the nature of those events and the external environment, that was at the heart of the problem. This made stress the problem of the individual, not of the organisation, institution or society, thus avoiding wider responsibility for any socio-economic circumstances which might be the cause of such suffering.

One solution the individual could access was a self-help book. Most of these books, in the first half of the century, were written for and about a middle-class readership, for whom problems of nerves and nervousness were linked to ideas of greater sensitivity and refinement that in turn were the preserve of the educated, professional classes. Overtaxing the brain through overwork linked stress to employment, but also to particular categories of employment that implied status. This can also be seen in the tendency in the later twentieth century to privilege executive stress and in the development of the stress management industry, which in the 1980s particularly tended to focus its attention on the senior ranks of white-collar employees. Gender also problematised stress in several ways. For most of the century, the world of work was understood as largely a male domain, despite the growing presence of women. Beliefs about work continued to privilege notions of masculine perseverance and toughness, even when by the end of the century, considerable shifts had occurred in gender roles and in psychological interpretations of work and its effects. As James Lyon's account suggests, for many men of his generation, it was a case of simply not recognising their own stress because the concept did not fit with their view of the world, work and themselves.

The specifically female version of nerves identified by Flora Klickmann in her interwar self-help book arose from the domestic challenges facing women who had 'no official working hours', and whose 'business premises never close'. Although Klickmann was largely referring to the work of the middle-class housewife, supervising others within the home rather than performing physical labour herself, she identified the home as a site of never-ending labour for women, while offering an escape from work for other members of the household.[6] For some women, the challenge of running a home, whether with help or alone, in the new suburban developments rapidly appearing in the interwar and post-Second World War periods, was understood as the cause of a specifically female form of stress, labelled suburban neurosis.[7] Very often linked to concerns about social mobility, increased privacy and the growth of consumerism, it was also grounded in an understanding of class and gender that saw women as particularly vulnerable to neuroticism created by housework and an over-enthusiastic pride in the appearance of the home that was rooted in social ambition. It was perhaps this latter, coupled with the rapid development of the post-war consumer society, that accounted for the longevity of suburban neurosis, which continued to influence researchers well into the 1970s, despite earlier findings that refuted its basis.[8]

Organisational attitudes towards the mental health of workers tended to be instrumental throughout the century. Early research in the interwar period focused on trying to identify susceptible workers, and this categorisation continued in the post-Second World War period, evidenced in publications aimed at those responsible for recruiting and dealing with workers. Such categorisation could be understood as a way for employers to focus their welfare efforts on stressed workers but was more likely used as a recruitment tool to avoid the employment of such individuals in the first place. Support for workers suffering from 'industrial neurosis', which led to the creation of Roffey Park Rehabilitation Centre during the war, was provided simply to get them back to productive working as soon as possible. Wartime demands meant that workplace stress was effectively validated, but it was a contingent validation driven by necessity rather than a real recognition of the effects of the workplace and working conditions on mental health. Arguably, it was the increasing threat of financial repercussions, partly through lost time but also in the face of successful prosecutions under the Health and Safety Act that eventually drove organisations in the late 1980s and 1990s to make more concrete provisions for dealing with employee stress.

Another factor influencing the increased organisational focus on stress in the last decades of the century was the considerable and visible public discourse that developed from the 1960s onwards and had become particularly significant by the 1980s. This came about partly through the opening to scrutiny of areas of life that had previously been seen as private but also because of an increasing focus in the media on health and ill-health stories. The 1960s and 1970s can be understood as the period in which popular ideas about who was likely to suffer from stress changed from a small elite of business executives and suburban neurotic housewives to almost anyone of any class and gender.

What also emerged from the increased public discourse, and particularly from newspapers, were continuing attempts to categorise

people and types of stress. Thus, the idea of burn-out became popularised, often associated with high-status executives but also with
specific populations within the public sector. This seemed to be a return
to privileging certain types of stress based on status, with City executives
equating to the 'brain workers' of the interwar period. However, the
fact that burn-out was also associated with teachers, nurses, doctors
and social workers also reflected the considerable turmoil and change
that these professions were undergoing during the period, as successive
governments attempted to cut the cost of the public sector. What is
very apparent from MOP accounts of the late century is that stress
was understood as the likely outcome of many situations and the
explanation for a range of experiences and suffering. However, while
greater awareness meant it might more easily be recognised and
acknowledged by the end of the century, ways of managing it and
treating it, despite the rise of the stress management industry, had not
changed significantly from many of the ideas offered in the self-help
books of the early century. What had changed was that the apparent
number and range of the stressed had expanded enormously, so that
in many ways by the end of the twentieth century everyone was stressed.

Lastly, I want to say something about the function that stress and
its precursors have served. I have already discussed the way in which
these concepts and the language used to express them incorporated
a wide variety of different experiences, and a multiplicity of meanings.
My analysis of self-help books argued that such was the breadth of the
symptoms, causes and explanations provided, almost anyone might
find them applicable to their own situation. Although this was obviously
inherent in ensuring a large audience when writing a popular self-help
book, evidence elsewhere supports the fact that this was not just a
marketing strategy. A catch-all label for a wide range of experiences
involving negative emotional responses to the troubles of life was, and
is, hugely useful. It was useful to the person who needed a description
for their bad experiences at work, but did not want to be medically
diagnosed and risk the loss of that employment; it was useful to the
busy GP who needed to acknowledge a patient's concerns and symptoms
without the necessity for a detailed diagnosis, which certainly explains
why neurasthenia was still being diagnosed in the 1950s and still listed
in the DSM in 1968; it was useful to the manager who wanted to
classify a range of sub-optimal workers; and it was useful to the

housewife unhappy in the face of apparently improved material domestic circumstances, fighting an often unspoken marital battle over roles and responsibilities and trapped within the confines of a suburban home.[9] An imprecise and flexible label that could be interpreted individually within a broad conceptual framework provided people with a way of categorising their own experience, without necessarily medicalising it in the way that a formal psychiatric diagnosis might. Such labels were useful shorthand because they provided an explanation of an experience, but at the same time left it undefined. Arguably this was empowering for the individual as they decided what constituted their suffering. Nerves and stress gave validity to people's experiences in a world that valued medical diagnoses without having to be too explicit about what they actually meant. The imprecision of stress and its lack of clear definition have enabled its appropriation by many different research disciplines and institutional stakeholders and arguably contributed both to its longevity and, by the end of the twentieth century, its ubiquity. Stress has not only captured the experience of the troubles of life, but it has encompassed concerns about modernity, change, technology, gender roles and class.

In the twenty-first century, stress continues to be frequently framed as an unresolved problem, the UN making workplace stress the focus of its World Day for Safety and Health at Work in 2016.[10] Stress is now understood as an international health problem, requiring policymaking and research tracking at a global level. How work-related stress is perceived, as this book has shown for Britain, depends largely on the kind of work culture that exists, and this varies from country to country. While newspapers in Britain continue to feature articles on how to tackle stress, repeating much the same remedies that featured in the self-help books of Chapter 1, governments in other countries have perceived and approached the problem in different ways.[11] As the *Guardian* reported at the end of 2016, new legislation in France meant that from 1 January 2017 organisations with more than fifty workers were required to negotiate with employees over the 'right to disconnect' from technology in an attempt to redraw the boundaries between work and home life, the blurring of which was considered damaging to employee health.[12] Evidently, for the French, technology and the encroaching of work activities into personal time were seen as contributing to stress. In Autumn 2017, the University and College Union, representing employees in Further and Higher Education in Britain, reported a case of a college lecturer successfully suing her employer for causing her stress, suggesting that despite widespread awareness of stress, organisations were still failing to comply with the Health and Safety legislation that held them to account for the mental as well as physical well-being of employees.[13] However, such legal cases were the exception rather than the rule, and for most stressed employees legal recourse was simply not an option. These examples indicate that, despite sceptical views in the late twentieth century, suggesting that stress was simply another fashionable concept waiting to be replaced by something 'more exciting', stress has continued to expand its reach, affecting more and more people to become a permanent feature of everyday life.[14]

Notes

1 James Lyon, Lives in the Oil Industry, 13 October 2003, C963/142, British Library Sound Archive.
2 *People in Production*, p. 257.
3 Lutz, 'Neurasthenia', 542; Busfield, *Men, Women and Madness*, pp. 190–1.
4 For example, Oppenheim, *Shattered Nerves*. Although there is considerable discussion of neurasthenia and nervous breakdown and Oppenheim makes similar arguments to mine about the multivalence of certain medical diagnoses and the cultural and social drives behind their popularity, specifically depression, somewhat surprisingly, she does not even mention stress.
5 Callahan and Berrios, *Reinventing Depression*, pp. 3, 30.
6 Klickmann, *Mending Your Nerves*, p. 48.
7 Taylor, 'Suburban Neurosis'.
8 Ineichen, 'Neurotic Wives'; Chave, 'Mental Health'.
9 Shorter, *Depressed*, p. 44.
10 'Workplace Stress "a Collective Challenge" as Work–Life Boundaries Become Blurred', UN News Service Section, 28 April 2016, www.un.org/apps/news/story.asp?NewsID=53807#.Wjk4fGhl-Ul. Accessed 19 December 2017.
11 'Seven Secrets to Becoming Stress Free', *Daily Mirror* (3 May 2016), p. 32.
12 'French Workers Win Legal Right to Avoid Checking Work Email Out-of-Hours', *Guardian* (31 December 2016), www. theguardian.com/

money/2016/dec/31/french-workers-win-legal-right-to-avoid-checking-work-email-out-of-hours. Accessed 8 May 2019.

13 'Art Lecturer Awarded £159,000 Damages in Bradford College Stress Case', UCU – University and College Union, 27 September 2017, www.ucu.org.uk/article/8948/Art-lecturer-awarded-159000-damages-in-Bradford-College-stress-case. Accessed 15 February 2018.

14 Doublet, *Stress Myth*, p. 86.

Bibliography

Unpublished primary sources

British Library Sound Archive

Mills, Jeff. Millennium Memory Bank Collection, 12 September 1998, C900/05537 © BBC.

Allen, Peter. Millennium Memory Bank Collection, 11 October 1998, C900/07016 © BBC.

Duckworth, Ken. Mental Health Testimony Archive, 11 March 1999, C905/21/01.

Lyon, James. Lives in the Oil Industry, 13 October 2003, C963/142.

Lloyds Banking Group Archive

Cullum, T. F. H. 'Note for Mr R. R. Amos, Deputy Chief General Manager' (28 July 1983), HO/GM/Off/213.

'Stress – Support, Not Survey', *Frontrunner*, March 1998.

'Well Said, and Thank You from All of Us!' *Frontrunner*, May 1998.

'Response to Last Month's Letter from a TSB Business Banking Manager Concerning Stress at Work', *Frontrunner*, June 1998.

'Some Tender Loving Care for Staff', *Frontrunner*, December 1999.

Mass Observation Archive, University of Sussex

Replies to directives

12 May Day Survey, 1937.

April directive 'Housework', 1951.

Summer directive 'Work', 1983.

Spring directive 'Social Well-Being', 1984.

Spring directive 'You and the NHS', 1997.

Summer directive 'Doing a Job', 1997.
Autumn directive 'Staying Well and Everyday Life', 1998.

File reports
FR 428, Report of Press Advertisements and Air Raids, 29 September 1940.
FR R520, Women and Morale, 10 December 1940.
FR 739, Preliminary Report: Questionnaire on Psychological War Work and
    on Air-Raids, 4 May 1941.
FR 926, Summary of Talk to the British Psychological Society, 26 October 1941.
FR 629, Health Questionnaire, 24 March 1943.
FR 1616, Some Psychological Factors in Home-Building, March 1943.
FR 2059, Will the Factory Girls Want to Stay Put or Go Home? March 1944.
FR 2285, Women's Reasons for Having Small Families, September 1945.
FR 2495, The State of Matrimony, June 1947.
FR 3110, General Attitudes to Sex, April 1949.

Diaries
D5284, Diary for 6 November 1941.
D5284, Diary for 7 November 1941.
D5311, Diary for 4 September 1943.
D5284, Diary for 5 November 1944.
D5284, Diary for 10 November 1944.
D5284, Diary for 8 December 1944.
D5284, Letter to Mass Observation, 4 March 1942.
D5284, Letter to Mass Observation, 4 February 1943.

Papers of Miss Richmond
Annual Report of Visits Made by Welfare Visitor (1945), January 1946.
Welfare Visitor's Report, 22 September 1949.
Welfare Visitor's Report, 24 May 1954.

The National Archives
Gray, P. G. 'The Housing Waiting Lists (England and Wales): An Inquiry
    Carried out in July 1949 for the Ministry of Health.'
'Civil Service College Annual Report and Accounts', Cabinet Office, April 1984.

Wellcome Collection
Central Council for Health Education in association with Scottish Council
    for Health Education, 'Just Nerves!' c.1943.
National Council for the Rehabilitation of Industrial Workers, 'Roffey Park
    Rehabilitation Centre: A Record of Two Years' Progress, 1944–1946', 1946.

Roffey Park Institute Ltd, 'Health and Human Relations in Industry: The Courses at Roffey Park', 1947.
Vernon, C. Harold. 'Confidential Letter to Hon. Arthur Howard', 1948, Roffey Park Rehabilitation Centre correspondence, memoranda and minutes of meetings 1948–49.
Roffey Park Rehabilitation Centre Advisory Panel, 'Confidential Report of the Advisory Panel Appointed by the Governors of St Thomas' Hospital in Connection with Roffey Park Rehabilitation Centre', 1949.

Published sources

Newspapers

Daily Mirror
'Peace-Time Prices', 19 February 1940.
'Collecting Fares in the Blackout Had Its Effect on Me: Trolley Bus Conductor Is Now "as Fit as Ever" Thanks to Yeast-Vite', 27 August 1940.
'You'll Stop Nagging Once You've Bought a Tin of "Peace-Time Sleep" Cadbury's Bourn-Vita Still at "Fear!"', 18 September 1940.
'When You Are "All Nerves": The Result of Worry and Anxiety Dr Williams Pink Pills', 29 November 1940.
'Keep Pools a Hobby – Not Worry Says Doctor', 31 December 1953.
'Drugs – Are They a Help or a Menace?' 19 September 1955.
'Secrets of the Pill-Takers', 20 September 1955.
'The Boss and the Deadly 10lb', 25 November 1960.
'The Fright of Our Lives', 10 October 1961.
'A Winner All the Way', 13 April 1962.
'The Rare Bird', 7 May 1962.
'"X" Film Show at Commons', 30 May 1962.
'"Early Warning" Plan for Swots', 16 July 1963.
'Advice on Problems of Middle-Age', 14 June 1965.
'A Boss's Burden Begins at Home', 2 May 1968.
'The Seven Ages of Stress', 20 October 1972.
'Stress: The Big Danger to Your Health', 9 July 1976.
'Death on the Dole … the New Threat', 27 August 1980.
'Seven Secrets to Becoming Stress Free', 3 May 2016.

Guardian
'Letters to the Editor', 2 October 1954.
'Letters to the Editor', 5 October 1954.

'Letters to the Editor', 11 October 1954.
'Letters to the Editor', 12 October 1954.
'Status Symbol of Stress and Strain', 16 March 1960.
'New Author and Old Outlook: The First Notable Alignment', 14 May 1962.
'Man "Broken by Stress"', 13 June 1974.
'When the Floundering Has to Stop', 10 October 1984.
'Study Finds Stress Hits Workers Most', 29 February 1988.
'Damages for Overwork', 17 November 1994.
'Phone Workers' "Brain Strain"', 6 January 1999.
'French Workers Win Legal Right to Avoid Checking Work Email Out-of-Hours', 31 December 2016.

The Independent
'Social Worker Wins £175,000 for Breakdowns', 27 April 1996.

The Observer
'Drama for the Millions', 22 April 1962.
'Stress Just Isn't British', 6 September 1998.

The Times
'All Our Own Work', 28 April 1962.
'Can Women Take the Pressure?' 17 February 1982.
'"Burn-out" Diagnosis on Hard-Pressed Doctors in NHS', 10 March 1984.
'Taking the Pain out of Strain', 24 January 1985.
'Working Can Be a Health Hazard', 24 February 1985.
'"Conspiracy of Silence" Is Blamed for Cost of Stress among Nurses', 2 May 1986.
'Stressing Pressures', 12 August 1987.
'Sir Calls It a Day as Pressure Builds', 25 October 1987.
'Concern at Teachers Quitting "burn-out" Careers', 1 June 1988.
'When the Going Gets Tough', 29 November 1990.
'One in Four Captains of Industry Wants to Jump Ship', 15 April 1991.
'Why the Office Is No Party', 28 October 1992.
'Unhappy High-Flyers and Housewives under Stress', 30 November 1994.
'Take Stress out of Success', 6 June 1996.

Television programmes
Kotcheff, Ted. 'Where I Live.' ABC for ITV, 1960.

Films

Jennings, Humphrey, and Harry Watt. *Britain Can Take It.* GPO Film Unit, 1940.

Reisz, Karel. *Saturday Night and Sunday Morning.* Woodfall Film Productions, 1960.

Richardson, Tony. *The Loneliness of the Long Distance Runner.* Woodfall Film Productions, 1962.

Schlesinger, John. *A Kind of Loving.* Vic Films Productions, 1962.

Books and articles

'A Rest From Industry.' *The Lancet* 246, 6376 (10 November 1945). https://doi.org/10.1016/S0140-6736(45)91627-8.

'A Specialist.' *From Terror to Triumph: How to Fight and Conquer Neurasthenia, Insomnia and Other Nervous Disorders.* Epsom: E. G. Pullinger, 1932.

Abrams, Lynn, and Callum G. Brown. *A History of Everyday Life in Twentieth-Century Scotland.* Edinburgh: Edinburgh University Press, 2010.

Alexander, Sally. 'Men's Fears and Women's Work: Responses to Unemployment in London Between the Wars.' *Gender & History* 12, 2 (2000). http://dx.doi.org/10.1111/1468-0424.00189.

Allport, Alan. *Demobbed: Coming Home after the Second World War.* New Haven; London: Yale University Press, 2009.

Alvarez, Walter C. *Live At Peace with Your Nerves.* Englewood Cliffs: Prentice-Hall, 1958.

An Enquiry into British War Production – A Report Prepared by Mass Observation for the Advertising Service Guild. Part 1: People in Production. London: John Murray, 1942.

An Enquiry into People's Homes: A Report Prepared by Mass Observation for the Advertising Service Guild. London: John Murray, 1943.

Ash, Edwin Lancelot Hopewell. *Nerves and the Nervous.* London: Mills & Boon, 1911.

———. *On Keeping Our Nerves in Order.* London: Mills & Boon, 1928.

———. *The Problem of Nervous Breakdown.* London: Mills & Boon, 1919.

Asher, Richard. *Nerves Explained: A Straightforward Guide to Nervous Illnesses.* London: Faber and Faber, 1957.

Barham, Peter. *Forgotten Lunatics of the Great War.* New Haven; London: Yale University Press, 2004.

Barton, Susan. *Working-Class Organisations and Popular Tourism, 1840–1970.* Manchester: Manchester University Press, 2005.

Baur, Nicole. 'Families, Stress and Mental Illness in Devon, 1940s to 1970s.' In Mark Jackson (ed.) *Stress in Post-War Britain, 1945–85.* Studies for the Society for the Social History of Medicine 23. London: Pickering & Chatto, 2015.

Becker, Dana. *One Nation Under Stress: The Trouble with Stress as an Idea.* Oxford: Oxford University Press, 2013.

———. *The Myth of Empowerment: Women and the Therapeutic Culture in America.* New York; London: New York University Press, 2005.

Bell, Melanie. *Femininity in the Frame: Women and 1950s British Popular Cinema.* London: IBTauris, 2010.

Bingham, Adrian. *Family Newspapers? Sex, Private Life and the British Popular Press 1918–1978.* Oxford: Oxford University Press, 2009.

———. 'The "K-Bomb": Social Surveys, the Popular Press, and British Sexual Culture in the 1940s and 1950s.' *The Journal of British Studies* 50, 1 (2011).

Bisch, Louis Edward. *Be Glad You're Neurotic.* New York: McGraw-Hill, 1936.

Bloome, D., Sheridan, D. and Street, B. 'Reading Mass Observation Writing: Theoretical and Methodological Issues in Researching in Mass Observation Archive.' *Mass Observation Archive Occasional Paper* 1 (University of Sussex), 1993.

Blunt, Alison, and Robyn Dowling. *Home.* Hoboken: Taylor and Francis, 2012.

BMA Special Committee. 'Medical Supervision of Industrial Workers.' *BMJ* II, 4221 (1941). https://doi.org/10.1136/bmj.2.4221.783.

Bornat, Joanna. 'A Second Take: Revisiting Interviews with a Different Purpose.' *Oral History* 31, 1 (2003). https://doi.org/10.2307/40179735.

Bornat, Joanna, Parvati Raghuram and Leroi Henry. 'Revisiting the Archives: A Case Study from the History of Geriatric Medicine.' *Sociological Research Online* 17, 2 (2012).

Bourke, Joanna. *Fear: A Cultural History.* London: Virago, 2005.

Braybon, Gail, and Penny Summerfield. *Out of the Cage: Women's Experiences in Two World Wars.* London: Pandora, 1987.

Brooke, Stephen. 'Living in "New Times": Historicizing 1980s Britain', *History Compass* 12, 1 (2014). https://doi.org/10.1111/hic3.12126.

Brown, Hilda. 'Some Effects of Shift Work on Social and Domestic Life.' *Yorkshire Bulletin of Economic and Social Research*, Occasional Paper No. 2 (1959).

Burnett, John. *Idle Hands: The Experience of Unemployment, 1750–1950.* London: Routledge, 1994.

Busfield, Joan. 'Class and Gender in Twentieth-Century British Psychiatry: Shell-Shock and Psychopathic Disorder.' *Clio Medica / The Wellcome Series in the History of Medicine* 73 (2004).

———. *Men, Women and Madness: Understanding Gender and Mental Disorder.* Basingstoke: Macmillan, 1996.

————. 'Mental Illness.' In Roger Cooter and John V Pickstone (eds) *Companion to Medicine in the Twentieth Century*. London: Routledge, 2003.

Calder, Angus. *The Myth of the Blitz*. London: Pimlico, 1992.

————. *The People's War: Britain 1939–45*. London: Pimlico, 1992.

Callahan, Christopher M., and German Elias Berrios. *Reinventing Depression: A History of the Treatment of Depression in Primary Care, 1940–2004*. Oxford: Oxford University Press, 2005.

Cannon, Walter Bradford. *Bodily Changes in Pain, Hunger, Fear and Rage: An Account of Recent Researches into the Function of Emotional Excitement*. New York; London: D. Appleton and Co., 1915.

Cantor, David, and Edmund Ramsden (eds). *Stress, Shock, and Adaptation in the Twentieth Century*. Rochester, NY: University of Rochester Press, 2014.

Carnegie, Dale. *How to Win Friends and Influence People*. New York: Simon & Schuster, 1937.

Chapman, James. 'Our Finest Hour Revisited: The Second World War in British Feature Films since 1945.' *Journal of Popular British Cinema* 1 (1998).

Chave, Sidney P. W. 'Mental Health in Harlow New Town.' *Journal of Psychosomatic Research* 10, 1 (1966). https://doi.org/10.1016/0022-3999(66)90134-6.

Clapson, Mark. *Invincible Green Suburbs, Brave New Towns: Social Change and Urban Dispersal in Postwar England*. Manchester: Manchester University Press, 1998.

————. *Suburban Century: Social Change and Urban Growth in England and the United States*. Oxford: Berg, 2003.

————. 'Working-Class Women's Experiences of Moving to New Housing Estates in England since 1919.' *Twentieth Century British History* 10, 3 (1999). https://doi.org/10.1093/tcbh/10.3.345.

Condrau, Flurin. 'The Patient's View Meets the Clinical Gaze.' *Social History of Medicine* 20, 3 (2007).

Conekin, Becky, Frank Mort and Chris Waters. *Moments of Modernity: Reconstructing Britain 1945–1964*. London: Rivers Oram Press, 1999.

Cooper, Cary L., and Philip Dewe. *Stress: A Brief History*. Oxford: Blackwell, 2004.

Cooper, Frederick. 'Medical Feminism, Working Mothers, and the Limits of Home: Finding a Balance between Self-Care and Other-Care in Cross-Cultural Debates about Health and Lifestyle, 1952–1956.' *Palgrave Communications* 2 (2016). https://doi.org/10.1057/palcomms.2016.42.

Crowther, Margaret Anne. *The Workhouse System, 1834–1929: The History of an English Social Institution*. London: Batsford Academic and Educational, 1981.

Culpin, Millais, and May Smith. 'The Nervous Temperament: Medical Research Council Report 61.' London: Industrial Health Research Board, 1930.

Currell, Sue. 'Depression and Recovery: Self-Help and America in the 1930s.' In David Bell and Joanne Hollows (eds) *Historicizing Lifestyle: Mediating Taste, Consumption and Identity from the 1900s to 1970s*. Aldershot: Ashgate Publishing Ltd, 2006.

Digby, Anne. *The Evolution of British General Practice, 1850–1948*. Oxford: Oxford University Press, 1999.

Doublet, Serge. *The Stress Myth*. Chesterfield, MO: Science & Humanities Press, 2000.

Durant, Ruth. *Watling: A Survey of Social Life on a New Housing Estate*. London: P. S. King & Son, 1939.

Ehrenreich, Barbara, and Deirdre English. *For Her Own Good: 150 Years of the Experts' Advice to Women*. Garden City, NY: Anchor Press, 1978.

Eisenberg, Philip, and Paul F. Lazarsfeld. 'The Psychological Effects of Unemployment.' *Psychological Bulletin* 35 (1938). http://dx.doi.org/10.1037/h0063426.

Endersby, Jim. *A Guinea Pig's History of Biology*. London: Arrow Books, 2007.

Feather, John. *A History of British Publishing*. London: Croom Helm, 1988.

Finch, Janet, and Penny Summerfield. 'Social Reconstruction and the Emergence of Companionate Marriage, 1945–59.' In David Clark (ed.) *Marriage, Domestic Life and Social Change: Writings for Jacqueline Burgoyne, 1944–88*. London: Routledge, 1991.

Fink, David Harold. *Release from Nervous Tension*. London: George Allen and Unwin Ltd, 1946.

Friedan, Betty. *The Feminine Mystique*. New York: W. W. Norton, 1963.

———. *The Feminine Mystique*. London: Penguin, 1965.

Füredi, Frank. *Therapy Culture: Cultivating Vulnerability in an Uncertain Age*. London; New York: Routledge, 2004.

Gallwey, April. 'The Rewards of Using Archival Oral Histories in Research: The Case of the Millennium Memory Bank.' *Oral History* 41, 1 (2013).

Garrison, Andrew. 'Restoring the Human in Humanistic Psychology.' *Journal of Humanistic Psychology* 41, 4 (2001).

Gavron, Hannah. *The Captive Wife: Conflicts of Housebound Mothers*. London: Routledge & Kegan Paul, 1966.

Gazeley, Ian, and Claire Langhamer. 'The Meanings of Happiness in Mass Observation's Bolton.' *History Workshop Journal* 1, 75 (2012). https://doi.org/10.1093/hwj/dbs015.

Giles, Judy. 'A Home of One's Own: Women and Domesticity in England 1918–1950.' *Women's Studies International Forum* 16, 3 (1993). https://doi.org/10.1016/0277-5395(93)90054-d.

———. 'Help for Housewives: Domestic Service and the Reconstruction of Domesticity in Britain, 1940–50.' *Women's History Review* 10, 2 (2001). https://doi.org/10.1080/09612020100200282.

———. 'Narratives of Gender, Class, and Modernity in Women's Memories of Mid Twentieth Century Britain.' *Signs* 28, 1 (2002). https://doi.org/10.1086/340907.

———. *The Parlour and the Suburb: Domestic Identities, Class, Femininity and Modernity*. Oxford: Berg, 2004.

Giles, W. John. *The First Forty: Roffey Park Institute 1946–1987*. Roffey Park Institute, 1988.

Gillett, Philip. *The British Working Class in Postwar Film*. Manchester: Manchester University Press, 2003.

Gillis, Stacey, and Joanne Hollows. *Feminism, Domesticity and Popular Culture*. New York; London: Routledge, 2009.

Goodman, Jordan. 'Pharmaceutical Industry.' In Roger Cooter and John V. Pickstone (eds) *Companion to Medicine in the Twentieth Century*. London: Routledge, 2003.

Grayzel, Susan R. *At Home and Under Fire: Air Raids and Culture in Britain from the Great War to the Blitz*. Cambridge; New York: Cambridge University Press, 2011.

Green, Francis, and Keith Whitfield. 'Employees' Experience of Work.' In William Arthur Brown, Alex Bryson and Keith Whitfield (eds) *The Evolution of the Modern Workplace*. Cambridge: Cambridge University Press, 2009.

Haggett, Ali. *A History of Male Psychological Disorders in Britain, 1945–1970*. Basingstoke: Palgrave Macmillan, 2015.

———. *Desperate Housewives, Neuroses and the Domestic Environment, 1945–1970*. London: Pickering & Chatto, 2012.

———. 'Gender, Stress and Alcohol Abuse in Post-War Britain.' In Mark Jackson (ed.) *Stress in Post-War Britain, 1945–85*. Studies for the Society for the Social History of Medicine 23. London: Pickering & Chatto, 2015.

Halliday, James L. 'Psychoneurosis as a Cause of Incapacity among Insured Persons.' *BMJ* 1 supplement 1584, 3870 (1935). https://doi.org/10.1136/bmj.1.3870.S85.

Harker, Ben. '"The Manchester Rambler": Ewan MacColl and the 1932 Mass Trespass.' *History Workshop Journal* 59, 1 (2005). https://doi.org/10.1093/hwj/dbi016.

Harris, Ben, and Courtney Stevens. 'From Rest Cure to Work Cure.' *Monitor on Psychology* 41, 5 (2010).

Harris, Henry Baruch. *How to Live With Your Nerves and Like It: A Family Doctor Book*. London: British Medical Association, 1956.

Harrisson, Tom. *Living through the Blitz*. London: Collins, 1976.

———. *War Factory: A Report by Mass Observation*. London: Gollancz, 1943.

Hayes, Nick. 'Did Manual Workers Want Industrial Welfare? Canteens, Latrines and Masculinity on British Building Sites 1918–1970.' *Journal of Social History* 35, 3 (2002). https://doi.org/jstor.org/stable/3790694.

Hayes, Sarah. 'Industrial Automation and Stress, c. 1945–79.' In Mark Jackson (ed.) *Stress in Post-War Britain, 1945–85*. Studies for the Society for the Social History of Medicine 23. London: Pickering & Chatto, 2015.

Haynes, Jo, and Demelza Jones. 'A Tale of Two Analyses: The Use of Archived Qualitative Data.' *Sociological Research Online* 17, 2 (2012).

Hayward, Rhodri. 'Busman's Stomach 1937: Digestive Disorders and the Making of Modern Politics.' *History of Emotions – Insights into Research* (2015). https://doi.org/DOI:10.14280/08241.36.

———. 'Desperate Housewives and Model Amoebae: The Invention of Suburban Neurosis in Inter-War Britain.' In Mark Jackson (ed.) *Health and the Modern Home*. New York: Routledge, 2007.

Hazelgrove, Jenny. *Spiritualism and British Society between the Wars*. Manchester: Manchester University Press, 2000.

Healy, David. *Let Them Eat Prozac*. New York; London: New York University Press, 2004.

Highmore, Ben. *Everyday Life and Cultural Theory: An Introduction*. London: Routledge, 2002.

Hill, John. 'From the "New Wave" to "Brit-Grit": Continuity and Difference in Working-Class Realism.' In Justine Ashby and Andrew Higson (eds) *British Cinema: Past and Present*. London: Routledge, 2000.

———. 'Working Class Realism and Sexual Reaction: Some Theses on the British "New Wave".' In James Curran and Vincent Porter (eds) *British Cinema History*. London: Weidenfeld and Nicholson, 1983.

Hinkle, Lawrence E. 'Stress and Disease: The Concept after 50 Years.' *Social Science & Medicine* 25, 6 (1987). https://doi.org/10.1016/0277-9536(87)90080-3.

Hinton, James. *The Mass Observers: A History, 1937–1949*. Oxford: Oxford University Press, 2013.

Hirshbein, Laura D. *American Melancholy: Constructions of Depression in the Twentieth Century*. New Brunswick; London: Rutgers University Press, 2009.

Hochschild, Arlie Russell. *The Managed Heart: Commercialization of Human Feeling*. London: University of California Press Ltd, 1983.

Hoffarth, Matthew J. 'The Making of Burnout: From Social Change to Self-Awareness in the Postwar United States, 1970–82.' *History of the Human Sciences* (2017). https://doi.org/10.1177/0952695117724929.

Horwitz, Allan V. *Anxiety: A Short History*. Johns Hopkins Biographies of Disease. Baltimore, MD: The Johns Hopkins University Press, 2013.

Hubback, Judith. *Wives Who Went to College*. London: William Heinemann, 1957.

Hubble, Nick. *Mass Observation and Everyday Life: Culture, History, Theory*. Basingstoke: Palgrave Macmillan, 2006.

Ineichen, Bernard. 'Neurotic Wives in a Modern Residential Suburb: A Sociological Profile.' *Social Science & Medicine* 9, 8–9 (1975). https://doi.org/10.1016/0037-7856(75)90077-3.

Jackson, Josephine A., and Helen M. Salisbury. *Outwitting Our Nerves: A Primer of Psychotherapy*. 3rd ed. London: Kegan Paul, Trench, Trubner, 1927.

Jackson, Mark. 'Stress in Post-War Britain: An Introduction.' In Mark Jackson (ed.) *Stress in Post-War Britain, 1945–85*. Studies for the Society for the Social History of Medicine 23. London: Pickering & Chatto, 2015.

———. *The Age of Stress: Science and the Search for Stability*. Oxford: Oxford University Press, 2013.

Jacobson, Edmund. *You Must Relax: A Practical Method of Reducing the Strains of Modern Living*. New York; London: McGraw-Hill Book Co., 1934.

Jahoda, Marie. 'Work, Employment, and Unemployment: Values, Theories, and Approaches in Social Research.' *American Psychologist* 36, 2 (1981). https://doi.org/10.1037/0003-066x.36.2.184.

James, Oliver. *Affluenza*. London: Vermilion, 2007.

———. *Britain on the Couch*. London: Century, 1997.

Jeffrey, Tom. *Mass Observation: A Short History*. Brighton: Mass Observation Archive, 1999.

Johnson, Paul. 'Introduction: Britain, 1900–1990.' In Paul Johnson (ed.) *Twentieth-Century Britain: Economic, Social and Cultural Change*. London; New York: Longman, 1997.

Johnston, Ronnie, and Arthur McIvor. 'Marginalising the Body at Work? Employers' Occupational Health Strategies and Occupational Medicine in Scotland c. 1930–1974.' *Social History of Medicine* 21, 1 (2008). https://doi.org/10.1093/shm/hkn003.

Jones, Edgar. *Shell Shock to PTSD: Military Psychiatry from 1900 to the Gulf War*. Hove, NY: Psychology Press, 2005.

———. '"The Gut War": Functional Somatic Disorders in the UK during the Second World War.' *History of the Human Sciences* 25, 5 (2012). https://doi.org/10.1177/0952695112466515.

Jones, Edgar, and Simon Wessely. 'War Syndromes: The Impact of Culture on Medically Unexplained Symptoms.' *Medical History* 49, 1 (2005). https://doi.org/10.1017/S0025727300008280.

Jones, Fiona, Jim Bright and Angela Clow. *Stress: Myth, Theory and Research.* Harlow; New York: Prentice Hall, 2001.

Jones, Helen. 'Employers' Welfare Schemes and Industrial Relations in Inter-War Britain.' *Business History* 25, 1 (1983). https://doi.org/10.1080/00076798300000005.

Kabat-Zinn, Jon. *Full Catastrophe Living: Using the Wisdom of Your Body and Mind to Face Stress, Pain and Illness.* New York: Delacorte Press, 1990.

Kendall, William Drummond. *The Conquest of Nerves.* London: St Clements Press, 1932.

Kennedy, John. *Relax and Live.* London: Prentice Hall, 1953.

———. *Worry: Its Cause and Cure.* London: The Psychologist, 1950.

Klickmann, Flora. *Mending Your Nerves.* London: RTS, 1925.

Kynaston, David. *Modernity Britain: Opening the Box, 1957–1959.* London; New York: Bloomsbury Publishing, 2013.

Laing, Stuart. *Representations of Working-Class Life 1957–1964.* Basingstoke: Macmillan, 1986.

Langhamer, Claire. *The English in Love: The Intimate Story of an Emotional Revolution.* Oxford: Oxford University Press, 2013.

———. '"Who the Hell Are Ordinary People?" Ordinariness as a Category of Historical Analysis.' *Transactions of the Royal Historical Society* 28 (2018).

———. *Women's Leisure in England, 1920–60.* Manchester: Manchester University Press, 2000.

Lay, Samantha. *British Social Realism: From Documentary to Brit-Grit.* London; New York: Wallflower, 2002.

Layard, Richard. *Happiness: Lessons from a New Science.* London: Penguin Group, 2005.

Lewis, Jane. *The End of Marriage? Individualism and Intimate Relations.* Cheltenham, UK; Northampton, MA: Edward Elgar, 2001.

Lewis, Jane, and Barbara Brookes. 'A Reassessment of the Work of the Peckham Health Centre, 1926–1951.' *Milbank Memorial Fund Quarterly: Health and Society* 61, 2 (1983). https://doi.org/10.2307/3349909.

Ling, Thomas M., J. A. Purser and E. W. Rees. 'Incidence and Treatment of Neurosis in Industry.' *BMJ* 2, 4671 (1950). https://doi.org/jstor.org/stable/25357681.

Long, Vicky. *The Rise and Fall of the Healthy Factory: The Politics of Industrial Health in Britain, 1914–60*. Basingstoke: Palgrave Macmillan, 2011.

Loosmore, William Charles. *Nerves and the Man: A Popular Psychological and Constructive Study of Nervous Breakdown*. London: John Murray, 1922.

Loughran, Tracey. 'Shell-Shock and Psychological Medicine in First World War Britain.' *Social History of Medicine* 22, 1 (2009). https://doi.org/10.1093/shm/hkn093.

Ludtke, Alf. 'What Is the History of Everyday Life and Who Are Its Practitioners?' In *The History of Everday Life: Reconstructing Historical Experiences and Ways of Life*, translated by William Templer. Princeton, NJ: Princeton University Press, 1995.

Lutz, Tom. *American Nervousness, 1903: An Anecdotal History*. Ithaca: Cornell University Press, 1991.

———. 'Neurasthenia and Fatigue Syndromes: Social Section.' In German Elias Berrios and Roy Porter (eds) *A History of Clinical Psychiatry: The Origin and History of Psychiatric Disorders*. London: The Athlone Press, 1995.

MacDougall King, Dougall. *Nerves and Personal Power: Some Principles of Psychology as Applied to Conduct and Health*. London: George Allen & Unwin, 1923.

Mackay, Robert. *Half the Battle: Civilian Morale in Britain during the Second World War*. Manchester; New York: Manchester University Press, 2002.

Mallett, Shelley. 'Understanding Home: A Critical Review of the Literature.' *The Sociological Review* 52, 1 (2004). https://doi.org/10.1111/j.1467-954X.2004.00442.x.

Marden, Orison Swett. *Making Friends with Our Nerves*. New York: T. Y. Crowell Co., 1925.

Markham, Miss Violet. 'Help for Housewives.' *The Listener*, 900 (1946).

Marwick, Arthur. 'Room at the Top, Saturday Night and Sunday Morning, and the "Cultural Revolution" in Britain.' *Journal of Contemporary History* 19, 1 (1984). https://doi.org/10.1177/002200948401900107.

———. 'The 1960s: Was There a "Cultural Revolution"?' *Contemporary Record* 2, 3 (1988). https://doi.org/10.1080/13619468808580986.

Maslach, Christina, Wilmar B. Schaufeli and Michael P. Leiter. 'Job Burnout.' *Annual Review of Psychology* 52, 1 (2001). https://doi.org/10.1146/annurev.psych.52.1.397.

Matthews, Jill Julius. 'They Had Such a Lot of Fun: The Women's League of Health and Beauty between the Wars.' *History Workshop Journal* 30, 1 (1990). https://doi.org/10.1093/hwj/30.1.22.

Maynard, Steven. 'Rough Work and Rugged Men: The Social Construction of Masculinity in Working-Class History.' *Labour / Le Travail* 23, Spring (1989). https://doi.org/10.2307/25143139.

Mayo, Elton. *The Human Problems of Industrial Civilisation*. New York: Macmillan, 1933.

McCarthy, Helen. 'Social Science and Married Women's Employment in Post-War Britain.' *Past & Present* 233, 1 (2016). https://doi.org/10.1093/pastj/gtw035.

McIvor, Arthur. 'Employers, the Government, and Industrial Fatigue in Britain, 1890–1918.' *British Journal of Industrial Medicine* 44, 11 (1987).

———. *Working Lives: Work in Britain since 1945*. Basingstoke: Palgrave Macmillan, 2013.

Melling, Joseph. 'Labouring Stress: Scientific Research, Trade Unions and Perceptions of Workplace Stress in Mid-Twentieth Century Britain.' In Mark Jackson (ed.) *Stress in Post-War Britain, 1945–85*. Studies for the Society for the Social History of Medicine 23. London: Pickering & Chatto, 2015.

———. 'Making Sense of Workplace Fear: The Role of Physicians, Psychiatrists, and Labor in Reforming Occupational Strain in Industrial Britain, ca. 1850–1970.' In David Cantor and Edmund Ramsden (eds) *Stress, Shock, and Adaptation in the Twentieth Century*. Rochester, NY: University of Rochester Press, 2014.

Merskey, Harold. 'Post-Traumatic Stress Disorder and Shell Shock: Clinical Section.' In German Elias Berrios and Roy Porter (eds) *A History of Clinical Psychiatry: The Origin and History of Psychiatric Disorders*. London: The Athlone Press, 1995.

Micale, Mark S. 'The Psychiatric Body.' In Roger Cooter and John V Pickstone (eds) *Companion to Medicine in the Twentieth Century*. London: Routledge, 2003.

Middleton, J. 'The Overpressure Epidemic of 1884 and the Culture of Nineteenth-Century Schooling.' *History of Education* 33, 4 (2004). https://doi.org/10.1080/0046760042000221808.

Miller, Ian. *A Modern History of the Stomach: Gastric Illness, Medicine and British Society, 1800–1950*. London: Routledge, 2015.

———. 'The Mind and Stomach at War: Stress and Abdominal Illness in Britain c.1939–1945.' *Medical History* 54, 1 (2010).

Mitchell, Gillian A. M. 'Reassessing "the Generation Gap": Bill Hayley's 1957 Tour of Britain, Inter-Generational Relations and Attitudes to Rock 'n' Roll in the Late 1950s.' *Twentieth Century British History* (2013). https://doi.org/10.1093/tcbh/hwt013.

Moore-Colyer, R. J. 'From Great Wen to Toad Hall: Aspects of the Urban–Rural Divide in Inter-War Britain.' *Rural History* 10, 01 (1999). https://doi.org/10.1017/S0956793300001710.

Moynihan, Ray, Iona Heath, David Henry and Peter C Gotzsche. 'Selling Sickness: The Pharmaceutical Industry and Disease Mongering.' *BMJ* 324, 7342 (2002). https://doi.org/10.1136/bmj.324.7342.886.

Mumby, Frank Arthur, and Ian Norrie. *Mumby's Publishing and Bookselling in the 20th Century.* London: Bell & Hyman, 1982.

Neve, Michael. 'Public Views of Neurasthenia: Britain, 1880–1930.' In Marijke Gijswijt-Hofstra and Roy Porter (eds) *Cultures of Psychiatry and Mental Health Care in Postwar Britain and the Netherlands.* Clio Medica / The Wellcome Series in the History of Medicine 63. Amsterdam: Rodopi, 2001.

Newton, Tim, Jocelyn Handy and Stephen Fineman. *Managing Stress: Emotion and Power at Work.* London; Thousand Oaks: Sage Publications, 1995.

Noakes, Lucy. 'Gender, Grief, and Bereavement in Second World War Britain.' *Journal of War & Culture Studies* 8, 1 (2015). https://doi.org/10.1179/175 2628014Y.0000000016.

Noakes, Lucy, and Juliette Pattinson (eds). *British Cultural Memory and the Second World War.* London: Bloomsbury, 2014.

Nudelman, Franny. 'Beyond the Talking Cure.' In Joel Pfister and Nancy Schnog (eds) *Inventing the Psychological: Toward a Cultural History of Emotional Life in America.* New Haven; London: Yale University Press, 1997.

Nye, Robert A. 'The Evolution of the Concept of Medicalization in the Late Twentieth Century.' *Journal of the History of the Behavioral Sciences* 39, 2 (2003). https://doi.org/10.1002/jhbs.10108.

Offer, Avner. *The Challenge of Affluence.* Oxford: Oxford University Press, 2006.

Oppenheim, Janet. *'Shattered Nerves': Doctors, Patients, and Depression in Victorian England.* New York; Oxford: Oxford University Press, 1991.

Overy, Richard. *The Bombing War: Europe 1939–1945.* London: Allen Lane, 2013.

———. *The Morbid Age: Britain and the Crisis of Civilization 1919–1939.* London: Penguin, 2010.

Owen, Alex. 'Occultism and the "Modern" Self in Fin-de-Siecle Britain.' In Martin Daunton and Bernhard Rieger (eds) *Meanings of Modernity: Britain from the Late Victorian Era to World War II.* Oxford: Berg, 2001.

Palmer, Debbie. 'Cultural Change, Stress and Civil Servants' Occupational Health, c. 1967–85.' In Mark Jackson (ed.) *Stress in Post-War Britain, 1945–85.* Studies for the Society for the Social History of Medicine 23. London: Pickering & Chatto, 2015.

Parish, P. A. 'The Prescribing of Psychotropic Drugs in General Practice.' *Journal of the Royal College of General Practitioners* 92, supplement 4 (1971).

Patmore, Angela. *The Truth about Stress*. London: Atlantic, 2006.

Pearse, Innes H., and Lucy H. Crocker. *The Peckham Experiment: A Study in the Living Structure of Society*. London: George Allen and Unwin Ltd, 1943.

Peniston-Bird, Corinna, and Penny Summerfield. '"Hey, You're Dead!": The Multiple Uses of Humour in Representations of British National Defence in the Second World War.' *Journal of European Studies* 31, 123 (2001). https://doi.org/10.1177/004724410103112314.

Perilli, Patricia. 'Statistical Survey of the British Film Industry.' In *British Cinema History*, edited by James Curran and Vincent Porter. London: Weidenfeld and Nicholson, 1983.

Perkin, Harold. *The Rise of Professional Society: England since 1880*. London; New York: Routledge, 1993.

Perks, Rob. 'The Century Speaks: A Public History Partnership.' *Oral History* 29, 2 (2001). https://doi.org/10.2307/40179712.

Pierce, Rachel M. 'Marriage in the Fifties.' *The Sociological Review* 11, 2 (1963). https://doi.org/10.1111/j.1467-954X.1963.tb01232.x.

Pitkin, Walter Boughton. *Life Begins at Forty*. New York: McGraw-Hill, 1932.

———. *More Power to You! A Working Technique for Making the Most of Human Energy*. Garden City: Garden City Publishing Co., 1933.

Pollen, Annebella. 'Research Methodology in Mass Observation Past and Present: "Scientifically, about as Valuable as a Chimpanzee's Tea Party at the Zoo"?' *History Workshop Journal*, 75 (2013). https://doi.org/10.1093/hwj/dbs040.

Pollock, Kristian. 'On the Nature of Social Stress: Production of a Modern Mythology.' *Social Science & Medicine* 26 (1988). https://doi.org/10.1016/0277-9536(88)90404-2.

Porter, Dilwyn. '"City Slickers" in Perspective: The Daily Mirror, Its Readers and Their Money, 1960–2000.' *Media History* 9, 2 (2003). https://doi.org/10.1080/13688800306758.

Porter, Roy. *Madness: A Brief History*. Oxford: Oxford University Press, 2002.

———. *The Greatest Benefit to Mankind: A Medical History of Humanity from Antiquity to the Present*. London: Fontana Press, 1999.

———. 'The Patient's View: Doing Medical History from Below.' *Theory and Society* 14, 2 (1985).

Powell, Danny. *Studying British Cinema: The 1960s*. Leighton Buzzard: Auteur Publishing, 2009.

Powell, Milton R. *How to Train Your Nerves: A Manual of Nerve Training*. London: Lutterworth Press, 1926.

———. *The Safe Way to Sound Nerves by Rational Nature Cure Drugless Methods*. London: Lutterworth Press, 1926.

Priestley, J. B. *English Journey*. London: William Heinemann Ltd in association with Victor Gollancz Ltd, 1934.

Ramsden, Edmund. 'Stress in the City: Mental Health, Urban Planning, and the Social Sciences in the Postwar United States.' In David Cantor and Edmund Ramsden (eds) *Stress, Shock, and Adaptation in the Twentieth Century*. Rochester, NY: University of Rochester Press, 2014.

Rapp, Dean. 'The Reception of Freud by the British Press: General Interest and Literary Magazines, 1920–1925.' *Journal of the History of the Behavioral Sciences* 24, 2 (1988). https://doi.org/10.1002/1520-6696(198804)24:2<191::AID-JHBS2300240206>3.0.CO;2-X.

Reid, Fiona. *Broken Men: Shell Shock, Treatment and Recovery in Britain 1914–1930*. London and New York: Continuum, 2010.

Richard, Jeffrey. 'New Waves and Old Myths: British Cinema in the 1960s.' In Bart Moore-Gilbert and John Seed (eds) *Cultural Revolution? The Challenge of the Arts in the 1960s*. London: Routledge, 1992.

Richards, Graham. 'Britain on the Couch: The Popularization of Psychoanalysis in Britain 1918–1940.' *Science in Context* 13, 2 (2000). https://doi.org/10.1017/S0269889700003793.

Richardson, Pamela. 'From War to Peace: Families Adapting to Change.' In Mark Jackson (ed.) *Stress in Post-War Britain, 1945–85*. Studies for the Society for the Social History of Medicine 23. London: Pickering & Chatto, 2015.

Roberts, Elizabeth. *Women and Families: An Oral History, 1940–1970*. Oxford: Blackwell, 1995.

Roper, Michael. *Masculinity and the British Organisation Man since 1945*. Oxford: Oxford University Press, 1994.

——— . 'Slipping Out of View: Subjectivity and Emotion in Gender History.' *History Workshop Journal* 59, 1 (2005). https://doi.org/10.1093/hwj/dbi006.

Rorie, Ronald Arthur Baxter. *Do Something about Those Nerves*. London and New York: Wingate Baker, 1969.

Rose, Nikolas. 'Beyond Medicalisation.' *The Lancet* 369, February 24 (2007).

——— *Governing the Soul: The Shaping of the Private Self*. London: Free Association, 1999.

Rose, Sonya O. *Which People's War? National Identity and Citizenship in Wartime Britain 1939–1945*. Oxford: Oxford University Press, 2003.

Rowntree, Benjamin Seebohm, and G. R. Lavers. *English Life and Leisure: A Social Study*. London: Longmans, Green and Co., 1951.

Saleeby, C. W. *Worry: The Disease of the Age*. London; Paris; New York; Melbourne: Cassell & Co. Ltd, 1907.

Savage, Michael. *Identities and Social Change in Britain since 1940: The Politics of Method*. Oxford: Oxford University Press, 2010.

Sayers, Dorothy L. *The Unpleasantness at the Bellona Club*. London: Ernest Benn, 1928.

Schofield, Alfred Taylor. *Nerves in Disorder: A Plea for Rational Treatment*. New York; London: Funk & Wagnells, 1903.

———. *Nervousness: A Brief and Popular Review of the Moral Treatment of Disordered Nerves*. London: William Rider & Sons Ltd, 1910.

Schuster, David G. *Neurasthenic Nation: America's Search for Health, Happiness and Comfort, 1869–1920*. London: Rutgers University Press, 2011.

Sedgwick, Eve Kosofsky. 'Epidemics of the Will.' In Eve Kosofsky Sedgwick (ed.) *Tendencies*. London: Routledge, 1994.

Seldon, Anthony, and Daniel Collings. *Britain under Thatcher*. Seminar Studies in History. Harlow: Longman, 2000.

Selye, Hans. *The Stress of Life*. New York: McGraw-Hill, 1956.

Shafer, Stephen C. 'An Overview of the Working Classes in British Feature Film from the 1960s to the 1980s: From Class Consciousness to Marginalization.' *International Labor and Working-Class History*, 59 (2001). https://doi.org/10.2307/27672706.

Shephard, Ben. *A War of Nerves: Soldiers and Psychiatrists in the Twentieth Century*. Cambridge, MA: Harvard University Press, 2001.

Shorter, Edward. *A History of Psychiatry: From the Era of the Asylum to the Age of Prozac*. New York; Chichester: John Wiley & Sons, 1997.

———. *Before Prozac: The Troubled History of Mood Disorders in Psychiatry*. Oxford; New York: Oxford University Press, 2009.

———. *How Everyone Became Depressed: The Rise and Fall of the Nervous Breakdown*. Oxford: Oxford University Press, 2013.

Showalter, Elaine. *The Female Malady: Women, Madness, and English Culture, 1830–1980*. New York: Pantheon, 1985.

Shuttleworth, Sally. *The Mind of the Child: Child Development in Literature, Science, and Medicine, 1840–1900*. Oxford: Oxford University Press, 2010.

Smail, David. *The Nature of Unhappiness*. London: Robinson, 2001.

Smith, May. 'The Nervous Temperament.' *British Journal of Medical Psychology* 10, 2 (1930). https://doi.org/10.1111/j.2044-8341.1930.tb01014.x.

Smith, Richard. '"Please Never Let It Happen Again": Lessons on Unemployment from the 1930s.' *BMJ* 291, 26 October (1985).

Spigel, Lynn. 'The Domestic Economy of Television Viewing in Postwar America.' *Critical Studies in Mass Communication* 6, 4 (1989). https://doi.org/10.1080/15295038909366761.

Stanley, Jo. 'Involuntary Commemorations.' In T. G. Ashplant, Graham Dawson and Michael Roper (eds) *The Politics of War Memory and Commemoration*. London: Routledge, 2000.

Starker, Steven. 'Promises and Prescriptions: Self-Help Books in Mental Health and Medicine.' *American Journal of Health Promotion* 1, 2 (1986). https://doi.org/10.4278/0890-1171-1.2.19.

Stevenson, Iain. *Book Makers: British Publishing in the Twentieth Century*. London: The British Library, 2010.

Stewart, Donald. 'Industrial Medical Services in Great Britain: A Critical Survey.' *BMJ* II, 4221 (1941). https://doi.org/10.1136/bmj.2.4221.762.

'Suburban Neurosis Up to Date.' *The Lancet* 1, 18 January (1958). http://dx.doi.org/10.1016/S0140-6736(58)90739-6.

Summerfield, Derek. 'The Invention of Post-Traumatic Stress Disorder and the Social Usefulness of a Psychiatric Category.' *BMJ* 322 (2001).

Summerfield, Penny. 'Approaches to Women and Social Change in the Second World War.' In Brian Brivati and Helen Jones (eds) *What Difference Did the War Make?* London: Leicester University Press, 1993.

———. 'Divisions at Sea: Class, Gender, Race, and Nation in Maritime Films of the Second World War, 1939–60.' *Twentieth Century British History* (2011). https://doi.org/10.1093/tcbh/hwr001.

———. 'Mass Observation: Social Research or Social Movement.' *Journal of Contemporary History* 20, 3 (1985).

———. *Women Workers in the Second World War: Production and Patriarchy in Conflict*. London: Routledge, 1989.

Tamboukou, Maria. 'Writing Genealogies: An Exploration of Foucault's Strategies for Doing Research.' *Discourse: Studies in the Cultural Politics of Education* 20 (1999). https://doi.org/10.1080/0159630990200202.

Taylor, Frederick Winslow. *The Principles of Scientific Management*. New York; London: Harper, 1911.

Taylor, Stephen. 'The Suburban Neurosis.' *The Lancet* 231, 5978 (1938). https://doi.org/10.1016/S0140-6736(00)93869-8.

Tebbutt, Melanie. *Women's Talk? A Social History of 'Gossip' in Working-Class Neighbourhoods, 1880–1960*. Aldershot: Scolar Press, 1995.

Theriot, Nancy M. 'Negotiating Illness: Doctors, Patients, and Families in the Nineteenth Century.' *Journal of the History of the Behavioral Sciences* 37, 4 (2001). https://doi.org/10.1002/jhbs.1065.

Thomson, Mathew. 'Neurasthenia in Britain: An Overview.' In Marijke Gijswijt-Hofstra and Roy Porter (eds) *Cultures of Psychiatry and Mental Health Care in Postwar Britain and the Netherlands*. Clio Medica / The Wellcome Series in the History of Medicine. Amsterdam: Rodopi, 2001.

———. *Psychological Subjects: Identity, Culture, and Health in Twentieth-Century Britain*. Oxford: Oxford University Press, 2006.

———. *The Problem of Mental Deficiency: Eugenics, Democracy and Social Policy in Britain c. 1870–1959*. Oxford: Oxford University Press, 1998.

———. 'The Psychological Body.' In Roger Cooter and John V. Pickstone (eds) *Companion to Medicine in the Twentieth Century*. London: Routledge, 2003.

Titmuss, Richard Morris. *Problems of Social Policy*. London: H.M.S.O., 1950.

Todd, Selina. 'Class, Experience and Britain's Twentieth Century.' *Social History* 39, 4 (2014). https://doi.org/10.1080/03071022.2014.983680.

Todd, Selina, and Hilary Young. 'Baby-Boomers to "Beanstalkers".' *Cultural & Social History* 9, 3 (2012). https://doi.org/10.2752/1478004 12X13347542916747.

Tomlinson, Jim. 'Reconstructing Britain: Labour in Power 1945–1951.' In Nick Tiratsoo (ed.) *From Blitz to Blair: A New History of Britain since 1939*. London: Weidenfeld & Nicolson, 1997.

Tredgold, Roger F. *Human Relations in Modern Industry*. London: Duckworth, 1949.

———. *Human Relations in Modern Industry*. London: Gerald Duckworth & Co. Ltd, 1963.

Turney, Jon. *Frankenstein's Footsteps: Science, Genetics and Popular Culture*. New Haven: Yale University Press, 1998.

Valverde, Mariana. *Diseases of the Will: Alcohol and the Dilemmas of Freedom*. Cambridge: Cambridge University Press, 1998.

Viner, Russell. 'Putting Stress in Life: Hans Selye and the Making of Stress Theory.' *Social Studies of Science* 29, 3 (1999). https://doi.org/ 10.1177/030631299029003003.

Wainwright, David, and Michael Calnan. *Work Stress: The Making of a Modern Epidemic*. Buckingham: Open University Press, 2002.

Walton, George Lincoln. *Why Worry?* Philadelphia: London: J. B. Lippincott Co., 1908.

Waterson, P. E., C. W. Clegg, R. Bolden, K. Pepper, P. B. Warr and T. D. Wall. 'The Use and Effectiveness of Modern Manufacturing Practices: A Survey of UK Industry.' *International Journal of Production Research* 37, 10 (1999). https://doi.org/10.1080/002075499190761.

Watkins, Elizabeth Siegel. 'Stress and the American Vernacular.' In David Cantor and Edmund Ramsden (eds) *Stress, Shock, and Adaptation in the Twentieth Century*. Rochester, NY: University of Rochester Press, 2014.

Watson, George Lincoln. *Those Nerves*. New York: Simple Life Series, 1910.

Watters, Ethan. *Crazy Like Us: The Globalization of the American Psyche*. New York; London: Free Press, 2010.

Weekes, Claire. *Hope and Help for Your Nerves*. New York: Coward-McCann, 1963.

———. *Peace from Nervous Suffering*. London: Angus and Robertson, 1972.

———. *Self-Help for Your Nerves*. Sydney; London: Angus & Robertson Ltd, 1963.

———. *Self Help for Your Nerves*. London: Fontana, 1992.

Weindling, Paul. 'Linking Self Help and Medical Science: The Social History of Occupational Health.' In Paul Weindling (ed.) *The Social History of Occupational Health*. London: Sydney: Croom Helm, 1985.

White, Ernest. *Overcoming Fears and Worries*. Watford: C&A Simpson Ltd, 1945.

Whiteside, Noel. 'Counting the Cost – Sickness and Disability among Working People in the Era of Industrial Recession, 1920–39.' *Economic History Review* 40, 2 (1987).

Willis, Paul. 'Shop-Floor Culture, Masculinity and the Wage Form.' In John Clarke, Chas Critcher and Richard Johnson (eds) *Working-Class Culture: Studies in History and Theory*. London: Hutchinson & Co. Ltd, 1979.

Wilson, Elizabeth. *Only Half-Way to Paradise: Women in Postwar Britain, 1945–1968*. London: Tavistock, 1980.

Wolfe, Walter Beran. *Nervous Breakdown: Its Cause and Cure*. New York: Farrar & Rinehart, 1933.

Young, Allan. *The Harmony of Illusions: Inventing Post-Traumatic Stress Disorder*. Princeton; Chichester: Princeton University Press, 1995.

Young, Michael Dunlop, and Peter Willmott. *Family and Kinship in East London*. London: Routledge & Kegan Paul, 1957.

Websites

'Art Lecturer Awarded £159,000 Damages in Bradford College Stress Case.' UCU – University and College Union, 27 September 2017. www.ucu.org. uk/article/8948/Art-lecturer-awarded-159000-damages-in-Bradford-College-stress-case.

'British Academy of Film and Television Arts Awards Database', http://awards. bafta.org/.

'Divorces in England and Wales 2010.' Office for National Statistics, 8 December 2011. www.ons.gov.uk/peoplepopulationandcommunity/ birthsdeathsandmarriages/divorce/bulletins/divorcesinenglandandwales/ 2011-12-08.

'Our Heritage: Timeline.' Lloyds Banking Group, www.lloydsbankinggroup.
com/our-group/our-heritage/timeline/.

'Workplace Stress "a Collective Challenge" as Work-Life Boundaries Become
Blurred.' UN News Service Section, 28 April 2016. www.un.org/apps/
news/story.asp?NewsID=53807#.Wjk4fGhl-Ul.

Unpublished papers

Jackson, Mark. 'Am I Ill?' Illness Histories and Approaches Workshop, History
Department, King's College London, 2012.

Unpublished theses

Blyth, Max. 'A History of the Central Council for Health Education 1927–1968.'
PhD thesis, University of Oxford, 1987

Whelan, Christine B. 'Self-Help Books and the Quest for Self-Control in the
United States 1950–2000.' PhD thesis, University of Oxford, 2004.

Index

Note: books and literary works can be found under authors' names

EU authorised representative for GPSR:
Easy Access System Europe, Mustamäe tee 50,
10621 Tallinn, Estonia
gpsr.requests@easproject.com